BELOVED SON FELIX

BELOVED SON FELIX

COMING OF AGE IN THE RENAISSANCE

TRANSLATED AND INTRODUCED
BY SEÁN JENNETT

WITH A FOREWORD BY STEPHEN GREENBLATT

McNally Editions

New York

McNally Editions
134 Prince St.
New York, NY 10012

Printed in the United States of America

Originally published in 1961 by Frederick Muller, Ltd., London.

First McNally Editions paperback, 2026

ISBN: 978-1-961341-68-5
E-book: 978-1-961341-69-2

Design by Jonathan Lippincott

3 5 7 9 10 8 6 4 2

CONTENTS

FOREWORD

THE MAGICAL CHARM OF *BELOVED SON FELIX*

In the early 1950s the Dutch historian Jacques Presser came up with the term "ego-documents" to describe the traces that people leave of themselves, whether in letters, diaries, memoirs, and the like, or in the many less formal ways in which the self makes itself known in the world. Though from the Early Modern period there are vast numbers of these traces, ranging from signatures on wills to love sonnets to obscene graffiti that people scratched on outhouse walls, there are very few ego-documents remotely comparable to the personal journal left by the physician Felix Platter. Keeping diaries and writing autobiographies did not become a widespread practice until the mid-seventeenth century. But it is not merely the relative paucity of such documents from earlier periods that makes Platter's journal so unusual. It is its vividness, intimacy, candor, and charm that confer upon it an altogether rare and revealing character.

When he set out to record for posterity some key moments in his life, Felix Platter (1536–1614) was already well advanced in a long, distinguished career in medicine.

He was much sought after as a clinician, venerated as a teacher, and celebrated as a scientist, having made significant advances in a wide range of areas, including anatomy, the function of the lens and retina, and the nature of psychiatric diseases. But in recalling the scenes of his youth, he did something extraordinary: he set aside his years of experience and knowledge of the world, and recovered what it felt like to be a naïve, untested teenager venturing out into unfamiliar and often dangerous territory. He relied on careful notes and revised the diary that he had kept at the time, drawing as well upon his prodigious memory. The result reflects rare gifts of inexhaustible curiosity, sharp intelligence, and a canny eye for detail.

Some of these gifts Felix must have been born with; others must have been conferred upon him or at least sharpened by those around him, most notably by his remarkable father Thomas. Thomas had lifted himself out of poverty in rural Switzerland to become a leading humanist scholar, printer, and schoolmaster in Basel. Along the way he became a Protestant, and it may in part have been the Reformation's emphasis on self-examination that accounts for his unusual decision late in life to write an autobiography. He is likely to have encouraged his son Felix to consider doing the same. Felix in turn encouraged his younger half-brother Thomas— known as Thomas Platter the Younger—to keep a journal now famous for recording a visit to the Globe Theater in London in 1599 to see a performance of Shakespeare's Julius Caesar.

The relation between Catholics and Protestants is a constant preoccupation in Felix's journal, and for good reason: it was a matter of life and death. With his father's encouragement, Felix had early determined to become a physician, and the distinguished medical school at which he hoped to study was at Montpellier in France. But the authorities in Montpellier, as in most of the French kingdom, were Catholic, and they were determined to root out what they regarded as a dangerous and subversive heresy. When, with a few coins in his pocket and a few more sewn into his jacket, the sixteen-year-old Felix set out on October 3, 1552 to travel the roughly 450 miles from Basel to Montpellier, he was not only leaving behind his family, his friends, and his German language, he was also entering a land where the practice of his religious faith could be fatal.

The risk was brought home to him very quickly. As he entered Lyon, about halfway to his destination, Felix writes in his journal that he saw "a Christian who was being led out to be burnt outside the gate; he was in his shirt with a truss of straw fastened on his back." Significantly, the word Felix uses here is "Christian," not "Protestant" and, still less, "heretic." Later in the journal he uses the word "martyr" to describe such victims. His own Reformed convictions then are always perfectly clear, but he needed to exercise discretion. One day, he notes, a commission marched through the streets of Montpellier declaring, to the sound of a trumpet, that anyone who knew of heretics in their midst would have to denounce them or be themselves severely punished. That Felix was not denounced is testimony to his prudence.

His father was prudent, too, and made sure to lodge Felix not in a Catholic household in Montpellier but with a pharmacist named Catalan, who was a Marrano. Catalan and his family were also Catholics in name and to some extent at least in belief, but they also secretly maintained Jewish practices, which Felix details in his journal with his characteristic acuteness. He also records a telling conversation he had with Catalan. (The conversation was in Latin, which was the language that the German-speaking Felix and the French-speaking Catalan had in common.) They were sitting by the hearth, and Catalan asked Felix to read to him out of an old Latin Bible, one, Felix observed, "from which the New Testament was missing." When Felix read a passage against images and idols, Catalan was delighted: "He was a Maran, and loved idols no more than do the Jews; but he did not dare to declare so openly." The Protestant Felix and the Marrano Catalan shared their hostility to religious icons – and they also shared a sense of caution.

In a moving account, Felix recounts the death in January 1554 of Guillaume Dalençon, a former priest turned Protestant who had already been defrocked, mutilated, and imprisoned several months earlier. Accompanied by two others convicted of heresy, Dalençon was taken to the execution ground where a pyre had been constructed. At the pyre, Felix writes, "he sat down on a log and himself took off his clothes as far as his shirt, and arranged them beside him tidily, as though he would be putting them on again." He was tied to the stake, with books he had brought from Calvinist Geneva placed next to him, and then burned to death. Felix, who had stopped in Geneva on his way to Montpellier and had met Calvin in person, describes this ghastly spectacle in detail, along with a still more ghastly one on the following day when the next victim was slowly burned on straw dampened by rain.

Well aware that he could suffer the same fate, Felix seems nonetheless to have maintained a surprising equanimity, and not only in the face of these religious menaces. For a modern reader the whole world in which he lived seems saturated with horrors. Nearing Nantua, on his journey to Montpellier, Felix and his traveling companions saw bodies hanging from the trees. "The night came upon us as we descended the mountain," he writes, "and it became so dark that we only just missed bumping into a corpse that was hanging from a branch." A few days later, as they approached Lyon, "we saw several men hanging from gibbets and others exposed on wheels." And still further along, not far from Nîmes, they passed the execution ground in front of the town: "Pieces of human flesh hung from the olive trees, and this sight gave me a curious sensation."

A curious sensation indeed. How did he or anyone else in such circumstances stay sane? The answer in part is simply one of expectations. Though the events he recorded in his journal struck him as worthy of note, they were not exceptions to the rule. They were simply the way the world worked. Thus, settled in Montpellier, he describes the execution—for what crime he does not specify—of "a fine young man." The victim's severed head rolled across the floor. Then "the executioner cut off both legs and both arms, and arranged them on the scaffold with the head in the middle and left them there all night." In the morning, Felix writes, "he hung them on an olive tree outside the town and there they were left to rot."

The next entry in the journal is, "On the 25th of July we went to Gramont to collect plants." The jarring discontinuity, typical of the journal, tells us a great deal about life in the sixteenth century, as Felix experienced it. He observed with care, he took it all in, and he went on. He did so in pursuit of his particular interests—collecting plants was a lifelong passion of his, closely linked to medical research and practice—and with a certain cool detachment that served him particularly well in his professional training.

In addition to the lectures which he assiduously attended, Felix by his own account never missed a dissection. Some of these resembled performances—we still refer to anatomy "theaters"—in front of audiences that included young girls and even monks, as well as wealthy nobles and bourgeois gentlemen. But as the Church discouraged prying into the secrets that God had hidden within the body, available cadavers were few. Therefore, Felix and his fellow students resorted to digging up recently buried corpses. On the first such excursion, as he calls these illegal escapades in the graveyard outside the city walls, they were aided by a renegade monk. On others they had to be wary of guards who were prepared to shoot at them with crossbows. When they had somehow managed to drag the exhumed bodies inside through holes in the wall—"I remember that I scratched my nose as I went through" (90), Felix noted—they unwrapped the grave clothes and set to work. Among the bodies that they dissected in this way was a student whom they had all known. "The lungs were decomposed and stank horribly, despite the vinegar that we sprinkled on them."

If these adventures were the sum of the contents of Felix's journal, we would value it as precious testimony of how a gifted medical scientist managed, against all odds, to obtain the training he needed. But there are other qualities that make it precious and—despite its elements of *grand guignol*—delightful. Felix had an unusual narrative flair, as he amply demonstrates in the account of his narrow escape from thuggish robbers—"eating roasted chestnuts and black bread and drinking cheap wine"—whom he encounters in an inn. Or again his confusion when, at another inn, he does not understand the local customs: "The innkeeper's daughter tried to kiss me, but I would not have it, which caused a lot of laughter, for it is the custom in this country to welcome with a kiss." Or again when, still booted and spurred from an expedition, he attempts to dance: "As I turned, my spurs entangled themselves in her dress, and I fell full length on the floor."

Here, as in many of these anecdotes, Felix reveals his weaknesses and laughs at himself. Though he was quickly maturing, he was still something of a child. Like most young men and women in this period, he shared a bed with someone, and in his case not only for warmth. When, on Christmas Eve, his bedmate went to Midnight Mass and left him alone in the house, Felix was terrified. "I took a lamp and shut myself in my study, which was at the top of the house, and was a plain little closet lined with boards. I stayed there until they returned from mass, reading the comedy of *Amphytrion* in an old copy of Plautus."

Part of his charm is his unpretentiousness, to which he adds an extraordinary eye for ethnographic detail. On entering Montpellier, he writes, "we met a large number of the inhabitants, of the nobility and others, clothed in long white shirts, and walking about the streets, preceded by stringed instruments and banners." He does not leave the description at that: "They carried in their hands shells of silver full of sugared almonds, and struck upon them with spoons of the same metal, and offered their sweets to every pretty girl they found in their path." So too he notes the colored candles sold in the shops for Christmas Eve; or the mock battles on Shrove Tuesday, with oranges as artillery and baskets as shields, leaving the Place Notre-Dame strewn with debris; or the "stalks of fennel ornamented with little figures of sugar" carried in the procession at the graduation ceremony for the Doctor of Medicine degree.

To highlight various features of Felix's experience and his writing, I have treated them in isolation from one another, but a significant part of the journal's power and pleasure is their rapid conjunction. Consider these entries from a few weeks in January and February 1554: "It was on this occasion that I made my first attempt at dancing in the French manner . . . I asked my father to send me some strings for my lute . . . On Shrove Tuesday the doctors went about the town in masks, and attacked the townspeople with a hail of oranges . . . On the 2nd of February there was another anatomy session, the subject being a man . . . On the 10th a criminal was executed. He was beheaded on a scaffold, and his four limbs were cut off . . . Doctor Honoratus Castellanus began to lecture again . . ." The giddy effect is not merely an artifact of the journal form; it conveys the actual flavor of Felix's life, with its pleasures and its perils, its commitments and its distractions, its inexhaustible curiosity and its steady focus on the great profession that lay ahead and to which he was to make so significant a contribution.

Stephen Greenblatt
Boston, 2025

INTRODUCTION

Montpellier became an important town after the destruction of Maguelone in the eighth century, and part of its prosperity came to be founded on the import of spices and similar products. The therapeutic value of some of these was recognized and led to a study of their uses in medicine. Men learned in this study began to teach younger men, and organized schools developed. By the twelfth century the School of Medicine of Montpellier was already renowned, and students came to it from all over Europe. A school of law and a university were also founded.

Though other regions were proud of their schools—it would be the greater honour, Felix's father wrote to him, to take his doctorate in Basel rather than in Montpellier—the fame of Montpellier was great, and a man who had studied there was to be respected. It was this high reputation, no doubt, that made Thomas Platter strive to send his son there, to get the best possible education to fit him for the profession he had chosen.

In Felix Platter's time the School of Medicine occupied a building on the slope of a hill in the northern part of the town, in the quarter towards Nîmes. This building was known to the students as the College. An ancient building still on this site may have been the school that Felix knew;

it is now occupied by the School of Pharmacy, the School of Medicine having moved in 1795 to larger premises, in the former Benedictine monastery next to the cathedral.

In the sixteenth century Montpellier was a walled town, of modest size, but already spilling out beyond the walls into faubourgs. The walls were dismantled long ago, and their line is marked now by the encircling boulevards. Indeed, the medieval town is gone, and little remains of the Montpellier that Felix knew. Though in his day there was apparent peace within the country, discontent against religious oppression was growing rapidly. Because he was a foreigner and a student, Felix was safe as a protestant, provided he did not flaunt his beliefs, but he saw other protestants who did not enjoy such immunity hounded out and burned at the stake. Especially in Languedoc, and among the upper classes, the desire for reform was desperate, and turning towards violence, and not long after Felix left Montpellier the fires that burned the heretics ignited the holocaust of civil war. Montpellier became a stronghold of the protestants, frequently attacked, and whether from the ardour of their faith or the urgency of the need for defences, they tumbled down many of the notable buildings and every one of the churches, with the sole exception of the façade and nave of the present cathedral. In Montpellier and its environs some sixty churches were thus pillaged or destroyed, and many monasteries, presbyteries, and similar buildings vanished. With Catholics and protestants in turn in ascendancy, and each eager to lay their hands on whatever stone or other material might be available for defences, there was no chance that any building, once ruined or decayed, would ever rise again;

its substance went into walls and bastions, into towers and emplacements.

Felix Platter came to a town that was medieval in pattern, not only in its architecture, but also in its way of life, in its thought, its festivals, its work, its manners, its law, its punishments. The spirit of the Renaissance had entered it, certainly, and was to be found in the teaching of the university, and certainly in the School of Medicine, but it had done little to affect the lives of the townspeople. Most of the elaborate structure of medieval life was swept away, not by the advance of progress, but by the internecine bitterness of the religious struggle. The town to which Thomas came forty years later was quite different from the Montpellier that Felix remembered, different physically and mentally. All his landmarks were gone. Felix must have discussed his beloved Montpellier with this very junior brother who was about to go there, and have described it to him; but it was a Montpellier of the past. Thomas found nothing to correspond, except the perpetual fame of the School of Medicine.

A few remnants of the sixteenth-century town survive, but they are sparse and unexciting. There are two fragments of the medieval walls—the Tour de la Babotte and the Tour des Pins—the latter named from a group of pine-trees which, incredibly, grew for two hundred years out of the stones of the summit of the tower; but that was after Felix's day. Then these towers were nothing distinctive; they were merely two among many in a strong and handsomely arcaded circuit of towers and walls. The Tour des Pins now houses the town's archives, which are deficient in documents dating to the sixteenth century, no doubt because of the wars then, but also because much valuable material relating to Montpellier was lost in the nineteenth century when an exhibition was burned down.

A number of old houses are to be found in the streets of the older quarters, but these houses have been much changed. Rondelet's house, for example, in which he received Rabelais, when the latter came to study medicine in Montpellier in 1530, now contains efficient modern shops opening on to the busy Rue de la Loge. Nevertheless, the many deep and narrow streets between the wider modern thoroughfares—between the Rue Foch and the Rue Saint-Guilhem, for instance, or farther over, up to the Grand Rue, or on the hill in the university quarter—follow the same course as they did in the sixteenth century, and in general appearance must present a similar impression, though most of the buildings may be of the seventeenth century. These confined alleys, perhaps rough underfoot, often odorous, winding, climbing steeply up hills and turning at times into stairs, and always with the vertical perspective of a canyon, these were the streets of Felix Platter's Montpellier.

Many of these streets still bear names with which he must have been familiar; the names of others have been altered as a result of that misguided passion of the French municipal authorities for perpetuating local or national celebrities at street corners. For example, the present Rue Stanislas Digeon was once the Rue Criminel, and was all the better for it; the Rue Roucher was formerly the Rue Triperie Vieille, which had some meaning—and if tripe is no longer prepared or sold there, the inhabitants are not such as would turn up their noses at it; the people of the Rue Hirondelle may not have soared like swallows, but they lived in something aesthetically preferable to the Rue Vallat. The old names remain because they are cut in pleasant humanistic capitals into the quoins of the corners, while the new ones, which unfortunately have currency, are given on wretched and illegible cast-iron oval plates.

The most striking survival from the Middle Ages is the facade of the Benedictine church, which is now the cathedral, with its extraordinary, naïve, and primitive porch—a vaulted stone baldaquin supported by two high and immense steepletopped towers at one end and the church wall at the other, as though it had nothing to do with the church and had somehow survived from a previous structure. This curiosity is so odd, and so unlike the pink and crocketed cathedral of Basel, and so impossible to overlook, that it is astonishing that Felix Platter does not mention it; for it must, one might have thought, have struck him at least as forcibly as the two columns of the Roman theatre at Arles, which he thought immense, and which are not a twentieth of the size of the ponderous pillars that hold up the open vault of the cathedral porch at Montpellier as appropriately as a pair of giants sharing a toy umbrella.

Felix's father Thomas Platter was a man of exceptional persistence, endurance, and dour ability, who began life in the poorest circumstances and battled his way through oppression, civil disturbance, religious intolerance, and personal misfortune to become a respected citizen of Basel, head of an important school, and owner of a printing establishment, four houses, and a farm in the country. His achievements in education, as a man who by his teaching helped to bring the Renaissance to Switzerland and Germany, have attracted the attention of scholars. He was never a rich man, however. His most dependable sources of income were his school, for which he received a salary, and the boarders he took into his houses, who sometimes numbered as many as thirty-five. Some of these boarders became afterwards well known, or travelled abroad—Felix met them as far afield as Montpellier, Toulouse, and Paris.

Felix was an only son, and became an only child. If this appears to contradict the fact that he had a brother, the contradiction is rather of words than of circumstance. He had had three sisters, all born before he was, but all of them died early, two in infancy and the third at seventeen. Felix might himself have died of the plague, as his sisters did, when his father and mother contracted the disease, if he had not been sent to the house of Peter Gebwiler at Roetelen, a visit he mentions early in this story. Felix, happily named, was destined for good fortune. His father was intent on improving the position he had achieved for his family, and it was surely to this end, as it was to Felix's inclination, that it was decided that the boy should become a doctor. The practice of medicine implied dignity and respect, and if the competition was severe, it offered the possibility of high reward for a man of ability. Such considerations influenced the son as well as the father; and yet it is evident that Felix's devotion to his study, which he does not emphasize in his journal, was not governed solely by the promise of the future, but also by apprehension of the past. His father's frequent adjurations spurred him, but so too did his knowledge of the dreadful experiences his father had undergone. Felix knew that his presence in Montpellier was the direct result of his father's determined pursuit of education and security, which he equated, and in studying to achieve his doctorate Felix must have been aware that he was strengthening the defences of his family against the want and wretchedness from which his father's efforts had raised it.

He came to study medicine at a time when that study was abandoning the superstition and half-magic of the Middle Ages and was turning towards observation and rationalization, towards the creation of a science of healing. Galen, with his doctrine of the governing humours of the human body, remained the basis of the practice of medicine, as had been the case for thirteen hundred years, with any change a change for the worse, a corruption of the original useful premise; but in the sixteenth century Galen was being observed anew, and in the light of a different mental attitude. Vesalius at Padua had quite altered the conception of anatomy, and had turned it in the direction of modern science. All these things the young Felix would become aware of, and indeed he shows in his journal that he is aware of them. Medicine remained still, in our view, abysmally ignorant of the causes of disease and of the functions of the body in combating it, but the new spirit was in the air. The School of Montpellier was among the best of its time, and its professors were in the van of progress; they observed and they deduced, they made their diagnoses and their prognoses, and they were followed in everything they did by students full of a lively spirit of inquiry. The course of study ended in severe examinations, which must be passed successfully before the candidate could be allowed to practise as a physician or a surgeon; and these examinations included very long debates at which the candidate could be put through the hoop not only by professors and licentiates, but also by his fellow students.

A man's education was rounded off by a journey through foreign countries or to great cities. There was not enough money for Felix to go wandering afar, and in any case the impatience of his future father-in-law compelled some haste. His devious journey through France is nevertheless to be considered in the light of education, besides being travel for its own sake—for Felix loved to travel. He returned to Basel a complete man, ready to take his doctorate and to set up in practice in his own town.

It is to Felix that we owe our knowledge of the Platter family. His urge to have some of the history of the family recorded was the force behind his father's autobiography and behind the journals kept by Thomas, his brother, from his Montpellier days onwards. Felix's notes on his life, on his stay in Montpellier, arose from a natural bent, a predilection, for writing, rather than from any external compulsion; but perhaps there was also, if concealed, a parvenu desire to create a background for his family. He persuaded his father to put down on paper the story of his early life, which Felix must often have heard from his lips, and the elder Thomas completed his autobiography in 1572, when he was seventy-three years old. It was addressed to his '*lieber sun Felix*', for whose education he had sacrificed so much, and whose achievement was now his pride. It was certainly Felix, too, who caused the younger Thomas to keep a journal when he in turn went to Montpellier in 1595. And yet, curiously, Felix's own journal lay neglected, unedited and unarranged, for more than fifty years, and it was the younger Thomas who persuaded him, in 1612, to bring it out and put it in order.

Felix's redaction cannot, however, have changed the original journal fundamentally; for the innocence of the early part of his account of Montpellier, and his journey there, could only have been written by a boy; and the visible growth from boyhood to the high maturity of a bachelor of medicine cannot possibly have been a literary exercise of old age. The journal, then, reflects the immediate impressions of an inhabitant of Montpellier in the middle of the sixteenth century, a living and personal voice across four centuries of time.

One disappointment came to alloy the father's pride in his son: Felix had no children. He had married his Magdalena on his return from Montpellier, but no child arrived to comfort the old man with the knowledge that his family would continue. When Felix's mother died, his father promptly married a second time, at the age of seventy-three, and of this second marriage two sons and four daughters were born. The elder of the two sons was also called Thomas; the other, Nicholas, died in his youth.

The elder Thomas died when his latter-day children were still small, and it is probable that the whole family was taken by Felix under his wing. Certainly Thomas was. Thomas was thirty-eight years younger than Felix, and the relationship between the two must have been more like that of an uncle and nephew than of two brothers. Felix treated Thomas as his adoptive son, and took great care of his education. In due course he was sent to Montpellier to study medicine, as Felix had done before him; while Felix went there at the age of fifteen, however, Thomas did not go until his twentieth year was passed, so there was an interval of more than forty years between these two student brothers. There seems to have been no question of finding an exchange for Thomas; Felix was now a successful man, approaching his sixties, a childless man willing to lavish care upon this son who was his brother. He was prosperous and could support Thomas in Montpellier with no indication of the financial strain that had never been absent from his own mind. Life was very much easier for this child of what was in effect, if not in fact, the third generation, a child to whom the poverty of his father's beginnings was a story of long ago. Whatever Thomas did in Montpellier, and in his more extensive journeys after he had completed his studies there, he was conscious that he could rely upon the comfort and support of that eminent gentleman '*mein herr bruder*'. Thomas was never ungrateful: he was as dutiful as Felix had been, and in time made his mark, but he seems always to be a shadow of Felix, with neither the lovable character nor the spark of originality of the elder brother whose ability and achievement always dominated his life.

Felix Platter's career after leaving Montpellier was a progress of solid achievement that justified all those who had prophesied a notable future for the boy whose intelligence and application must have been obvious from his earliest days. He became the principal physician of the town, a professor and rector of the university, and attended the great of France and Switzerland. He worked with devotion and distinction in the periodic outbreaks of plague in the Basel district, and kept a close account of their ravages in a manuscript book that now lies in the library of the University of Basel. He built a very large and sumptuous house, which a contemporary describes as 'most painted and ornate, with arabesques in the French style'. Felix was eminently a successful bourgeois, and what, in Switzerland, could be more admirable? He had splendidly fulfilled his father's ambition for him. And yet, however eminent he might be, however fine his house, he was of the *petite bourgeoisie* and never forgot the penury of his childhood or the value of money, in sums however small. Another contemporary saw something of Felix's extensive collection of natural objects, a veritable museum, which he had begun as long ago as his days in Montpellier, when he had frequently sent home to Basel boxes full of a miscellany of things—dried crabs, lobsters, seashells, leaves of Indian fig-trees for planting, and so forth. It was augmented by many consignments from Thomas in his time in Montpellier. There were fossils to be seen, curious stones, and in the stable a wild ass and a marmot. This private museum was clearly well worth visiting, but no one saw it without first paying an entrance fee, and Felix meticulously set down the total of these fees in his accounts.

He enjoyed a long and useful life, and died in 1614. His wife Magdalena had died the year before.

Felix wrote various books and essays on medicine, setting out the knowledge and experience he had gained. It was not an uncommon practice for medical men to do this, and there was no extraordinary reputation to be obtained unless a man had something both right and revolutionary to say, like Vesalius in the first half of the sixteenth century or Harvey in the seventeenth. These works confirmed his position as a teacher and a physician.

Felix's brother, Thomas, had a son, born in 1605, who was called Felix after his uncle; this Felix in turn had a son, Franz, born in 1645. Franz died in 1711 without male issue, and so with him the direct line of the Platters came to an end.

Felix Platter's journal is valuable as an historical document because it describes the life of a period in Montpellier that is not otherwise well supplied with documents, and illustrates something of the manner and the system of medical education. If it did this and no more, it would have value; but it is more than a mere archive: it is also a work of literary interest, in its delightful revelation of the character of a young man faced at an impressionable age with the responsibilities of serious study and of independence in a foreign town, of whose language at first he was quite ignorant. Utterly honest and frank, at times timid, at times gay, Felix always enjoyed his life in Montpellier, and described with a delicate ingenuousness the frolics, the work, and the brutality of his time.

He was an inveterate hoarder, a preserver of old papers of the kind blessed by the historian. His museum is an example of his collecting instinct; yet another is his preservation of letters, so that we have collections of letters sent to him in Montpellier by his father, by Jacques and Gilbert Catalan, and others, as well as the volume of his journal;

and further, there is a fine herbal, full of plants pressed with the art that he learned in Montpellier. All these are in the library of the University of Basel.

The manuscript of the journal, like all the other material, is in excellent condition, and it is written in a careful and usually legible hand. It is in the dialect of German then current in Basel. Felix's journal was first published, in German, in 1840, preceded by his father's autobiography. There have been other editions from that time to the present day, some of the modem ones being very much abridged. The best edition is that edited by H. Boos and published in 1878. Those parts of the journal concerning Montpellier, with his journey there and back, were published in French, together with the corresponding part of the younger Thomas's journal, in a very limited edition (190 copies), pleasantly printed on large paper, by the Société des Bibliophiles de Montpellier in 1892. This edition contains numerous notes, and this, together with the Boos edition, has been used for the present translation into English.

Seán Jennett
1961

BELOVED SON FELIX

1

THE JOURNEY FROM BASEL TO MONTPELLIER

From my childhood I had always dreamed of studying medicine and of becoming a doctor. My father desired it as much as I did, for he had himself once approached the same study. He often spoke to me of the esteem that doctors enjoy, and when I was still a child he made me admire them as they passed on horseback in the street. Considering, then, that I had arrived at the age of fifteen, and that I was an only son, he resolved, that I might the sooner become a doctor, and in good time be a support for the family, to send me to Montpellier, where in those days the study of medicine flourished.

Some years before he had begun to seek an exchange for me, as Frederick Rihener had been exchanged with one of Catalan's sons. He hoped that I might be able to take the place of Rihener, who had already been three years in Montpellier. This hope was encouraged by Henry Volffius, brother of Jerome Volffius, who used to live in our house, and he had worked hard to arrange the matter with Catalan. He had been tutor to Catalan's children before

Rihener came to Montpellier. Rihener, too, had promised to do all he could, before he left, to arrange that I should take his place with Catalan. My father and I therefore waited with impatience for an opportunity; it was not long in coming.

Rihener, who was in Montpellier in exchange[1] with Jacob Catalan, who was in Basel with Rihener's father, went to live in Paris. His place with Catalan was taken by Jacob Meier of Strasbourg, and so Catalan's son left Basel to go to Meier's house in Strasbourg. His brother Gilbert Catalan was already in that town, in exchange for Johann Odratzheim, who was also with Catalan in Montpellier. As Odratzheim's studies were sufficiently well advanced to allow us to suppose that his departure would not be long delayed, my father, encouraged by these circumstances and by the letter of recommendation that Volffius had given us for Catalan, resolved to take a chance. It was the time of the autumn fair in Frankfurt, which the merchants of Lyon customarily attend. My father decided to take advantage of their return to Lyon to send me with them as far as that town. Thomas Schoepfius, a schoolmaster from Saint Peter's, also wished to go to Lyon, and this was fortunate, for my youth made it necessary that someone should take care of me.

My father bought a little horse for me for seven crowns. Unhappily the plague was abroad in the country, and we could not be sure that the merchants would come through Basel on their way to Lyon. We had counted especially on a man called Beringer, but he passed by without our knowledge, and so the merchants of Lyon proved of no benefit to us. Fortunately a Parisian arrived, on his way to

Geneva. He was a man of fine manners, called Robert. He stayed for a few days in Basel and then took us with him. We hoped that we should find in Geneva an opportunity to continue our journey. It had been in my father's mind, when the plague broke out, to send me either to Zurich or to Geneva.

On the 3rd of October, in the year 1552, I rode on my little horse to Roetelen, to the house of Doctor Peter Gebwiler, *greffier* of the canton, with whom I had stayed for a time, and took leave of him and his wife.

On the 9th of October, a Sunday, my father wrapped up two shirts and some handkerchiefs in a waxed cloth for me, and gave me three crowns in change. Four other crowns, in gold, he had taken the precaution to sew into my jerkin. He told me that he had borrowed the money, and also that required to pay for the horse. He made me a present of a Valaison thaler, struck under the cardinal Matthew Schinner: I brought it back to the house several years later. My mother also gave me a crown. Finally, my father gave me the most strict instructions: I must never presume on the fact that I was an only son, for although he had some property, he had many debts; I must study zealously in order to gain mastery of my art; and I must do all that I could to get in to Catalan's house as an exchange. He promised that in any case he would never abandon me.

At my father's invitation Meister Franz,[2] who later became my father-in-law, came to our last supper. This gave me great pleasure, for it made me believe that the arrangements for my marriage had been made. My mother had prepared a roast rabbit and a quail, which I had reared myself, and which she had killed on my account. She loved to tease, and she took advantage of a moment when Daniel Jeckelmann was making a show of lighting a lantern to take his father home, to say: 'Felix, sit beside Daniel, your future brother-in-law, perhaps'. I pretended not to have understood. Before the end of the supper someone came in great haste for Meister Franz to come and cure Batt Meier, who had felt the first symptoms of the plague. It was not yet nine o'clock, but he bade me farewell, wished me happiness, and left.

In the morning, the 10th of October, it was not until after nine o'clock that Thomas Schoepfius and our companion Robert appeared on horseback, and so it was already late by the time we were ready to depart. I said good-bye to my mother, who wept and thought that she would never see me again, considering the many years that I was to remain abroad. She also feared that Basel might be utterly destroyed by the army of Charles V, which was on its way to besiege Metz.[3]

We set off on the road. My father, who was going to accompany us part of the way, had gone to await us at Liechstal, two miles from Basel. There, as I descended a stair, I tripped over my spurs, to which I was not accustomed, and came near to falling from top to bottom. We dined at an inn, the *Key*, and the host, the father of Jacob Martin, who was a student at Basel, made me a present of the score. The day was advanced by the time we left. My father came with us as far as the chapel outside the gate. There he held out his hand to say good-bye and tried to say 'Felix, *vale*', but he could not utter the word *vale*; he could get only as far as va . . .', and he went away quite overcome. My heart was heavy and I continued sadly a journey to

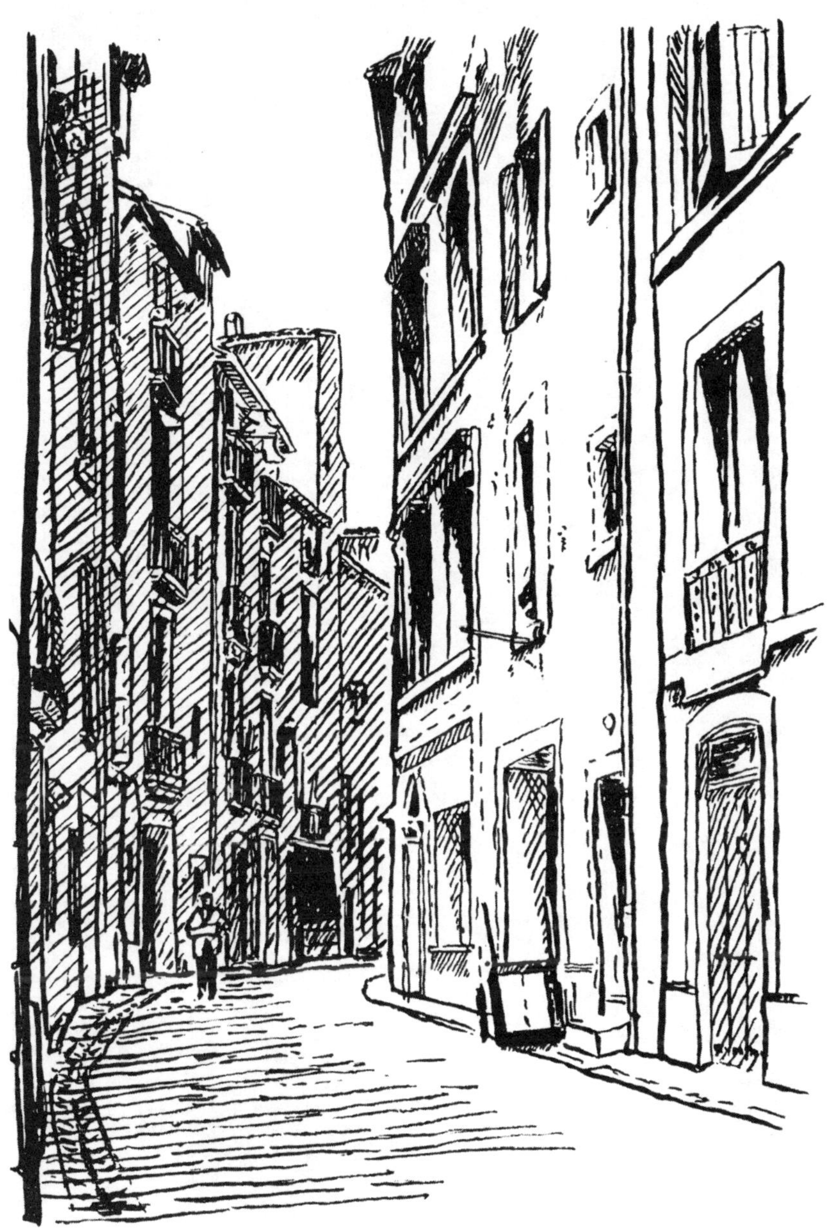

1. A Street in Montpellier (drawing by Seán Jennett)

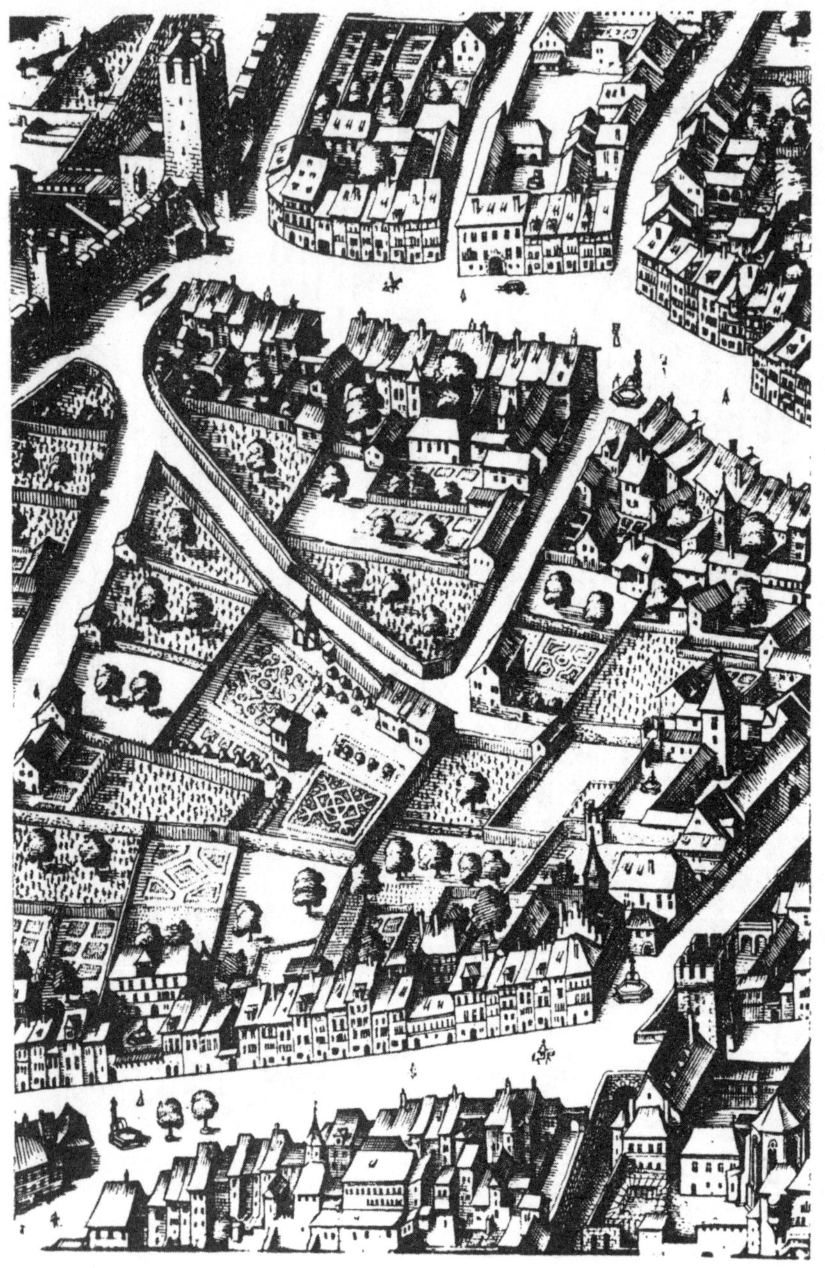

2. Aerial view of Basel, showing 'zum Gejegt', Thomas Platter's house—the large house with four dormers

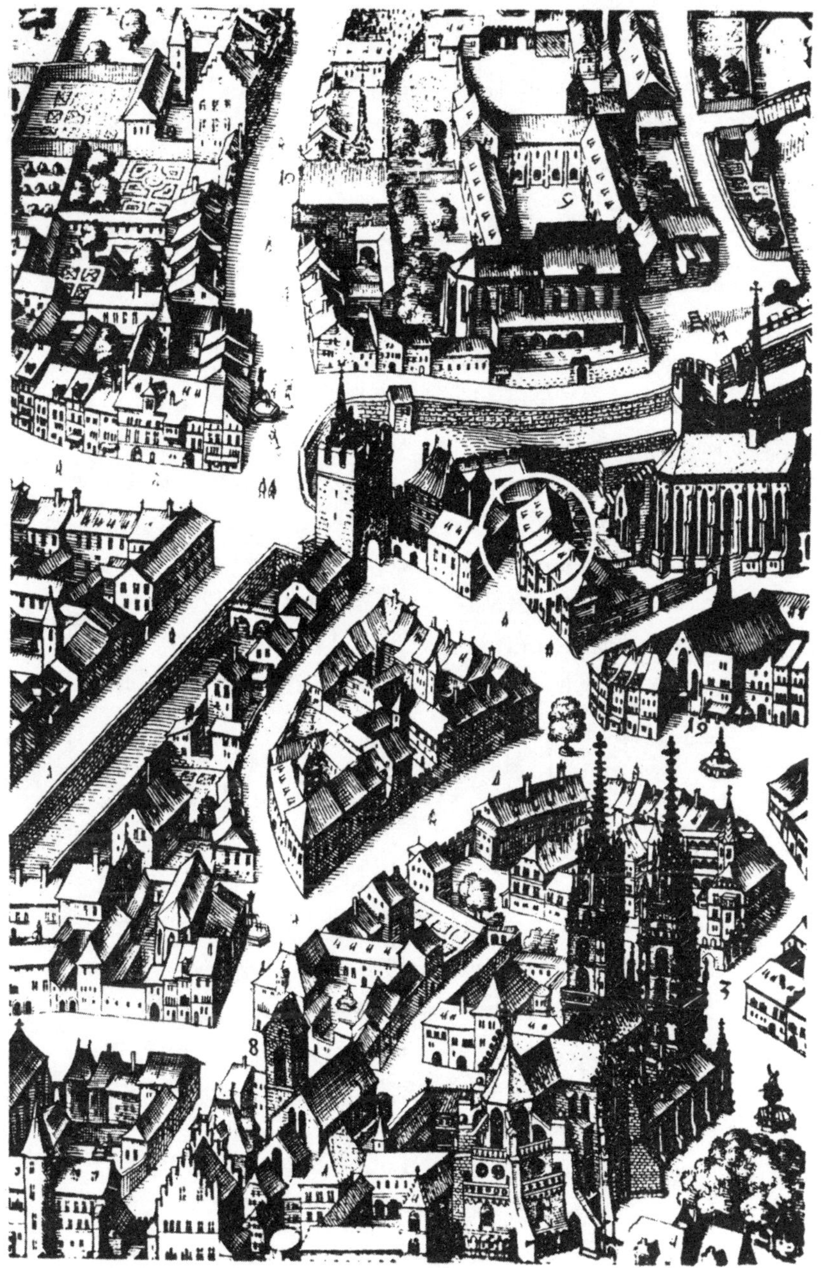

within the white circle. From a view of Basel engraved by Merian in 1615, in the Stadtsarchiv, Basel which I had so eagerly looked forward. My father wrote to me afterwards that on his return home he found our servant Anne sick with the plague, and that the servant of Thomas Schoepfius had been stricken the same day. He thanked God that we had left in time, before we should be exposed to the contagion, which was rife in Basel and in our street.

We arrived rather late in the little town of Waldenburg, a mile from Liechstal, but we resolved to push on to Balsthal. However, the night came upon us at Hauenstein, where my horse fell and threw me against a rock; but I was not hurt. We came to the village of Langenbruck, a mile from Waldenburg, and stopped at the *Horse*.

On the 11th of October we left for Balsthal, which is a mile[4] from Langenbruck, passed through the village of Wietlispach, and reached Solothurn, a mile beyond Balsthal. We dined at the *Lion*. It was the time of the fair. Master Georg, the organist, took us to the church and showed us the organ, on which my companion Thomas Schoepfius played a little. Late in the evening we passed the convent of Frauwbrunnen, two miles from Solothurn. Near there, in a field, we saw a stone column with this inscription on a plaque: '1375 years after the birth of Jesus Christ, the day of St. John of Christmas, the English, who are called Gigler, were, with the help of God, defeated and put to flight, in a hard combat, by the people of Bern.

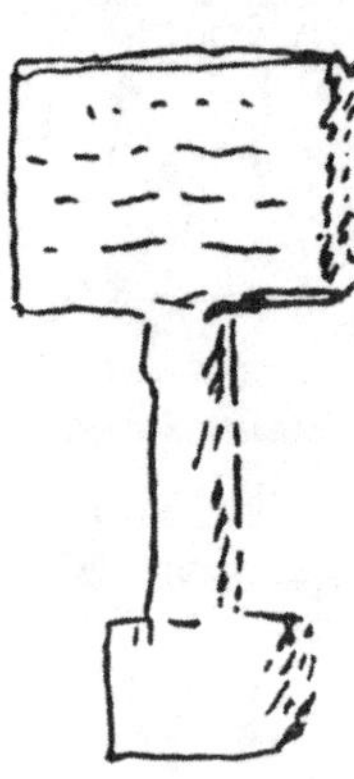

3. Felix Platter's drawing of the stone near Solothurn (tracing from the manuscript of the journal)

Praised be God for ever.'[5] It was already dusk and we could scarcely make out the inscription. Farther on, beyond a forest, we arrived in the village of Jagersdorf, where the night compelled us to stay. The inn was full of peasants, and the smoke stifled us all night.

On the 12th of October we arrived safely in Bern. We descended at the *Falcon*, and looked around the town and at the churches and the banners, and also at the bears—there were six of them in the pits. After midday we continued our journey. Passing over the bridge at Köniz, I drank from a pretty fountain. There we met a young couple, just married, who decided to come with us. While the young woman was jogging along beside me, and her husband with the others, she got caught in an apple tree, fell off her horse, and remained suspended on the tree, with all her skirts raised, until someone came to rescue her. Three miles from Bern, we reached Fribourg, where we stayed at the *White Cross*. It was there that we began to eat and to sleep in the French fashion.

On the 13th of October the weather changed and it began to rain, which annoyed me a great deal. We were soaked going through the French villages on the way to Romont. When we arrived at this place we stopped at the *Lion* to dry our clothes. After dinner we took the road to Lausanne. In the hamlet of Rue, Thomas lost us and we had to wait a long time until he found us again. The night came, with a thick mist, and we lost our way. We came into the forest of Jurthen, where it was not safe to travel at that time. We wanted nothing more than a barn, a shelter of some sort, to keep out of the rain. After wandering about for a long time we found a village, but were refused hospitality there. So we hired a young man to show us the way through the wood, and he led us to a place called Mézières.[6] There was a wretched inn there with a few houses scattered around it. It was kept by a woman, who could find space for us only on the ground floor, in a room open to all the four winds. In this room was a long table, at which sat a number of Savoyard peasants and beggars, eating roasted chestnuts and black bread and drinking cheap wine.

We would gladly have continued our journey if it had not been that we were wet through from the rain and the night was dark. We were obliged to stay, even though the woman declared that she had neither bed nor stable. We settled our horses as well as we could in a low and narrow stall, where they remained all night saddled and bridled. As for us, we had to sit down beside the rascals at the table and content ourselves with the same fare. We soon realized what kind of people we had to deal with, for they eyed our weapons and taunted us, though we took care not to give them cause for annoyance. They got drunk and went staggering out of the room to lie down beside the fire that still burned in the hearth in the next chamber. They soon fell asleep. It was this that saved us, for we learned next morning from our guide that they had intended to kill us; he had heard them plotting as he lay awake on the straw.

We too had been uneasy about them. We closed the shutters and pushed a broken bed against the door. Then, having set our naked rapiers on the table, we watched all night. I was a prey to all sorts of terrors, for I was young and had never travelled before. After we had gone a long time like this, Robert and Thomas agreed that it would be wise to take advantage of the men while they slept—we could hear them snoring—and, recommending ourselves to God, go quietly in search of our mounts, and leave in no matter what direction. We had already settled the account with the woman of the inn. Cautiously we pulled the old bed away from the door and went out. They were all asleep. We went to the stall and got out our horses, and as we did so the guide joined us. He told Robert, who was the only one of us who understood French, that the men had meant to rise early and wait for us in the forest, and there attack us. But we were leaving three hours before daylight, and they were still in a deep sleep, thanks be to God. We promised the guide a reward if he would lead us to Lausanne by a by-road, for we feared that other bandits might lie in wait for us on the main road. He led us through the wood, and when the dawn came, we rejoined the road, giving thanks to God.

Towards noon we came to Lausanne, which is three miles from Fribourg, and stopped at the *Ange*. We were soaked to the bone and drooping with weariness. Our horses were in no better state, for they had eaten nothing for twenty-four hours. We told people in Lausanne of the dangers we had been through, and when we mentioned the name of the place, they said that it was a wonder that we had not all been killed. Murders were committed daily in the forest of Jurthen by a band led by a man called Long Peter. Not long afterwards he was broken on the wheel in Bern, and among other confessions he declared that he had planned to kill some students at Mézières. Thomas learned this in Bern after his return from Montpellier, and told me of it in a letter.

After dinner we rode alongside the lake of Geneva as far as Morges, which is a mile from Lausanne, and afterwards to Rolle, which is two miles farther on, and here we passed the night at the *White Cross*. This inn is kept by a German.

On the 15th of October we set out for Geneva, along the lake and by way of Nyon and Coppet, and there we stayed at the *Lion*. After dinner we explored the town. As I had been teased frequently about my hair, which I had worn long since childhood, after the fashion of that time, I went first of all to have it cut very short. As a result I got catarrh, a complaint I had never had till then. I went to Meister Calvin's house and gave him a letter in which my father recommended Schoepfius and me to him. As soon as he had read it, he said: 'Master Felix, this is very convenient. I have an excellent travelling companion for you, a surgeon called Michel Heroardus, who is from Montpellier. He will leave tomorrow or the day after and you could not wish for a better companion.' This news was all the more agreeable because Robert was going to remain in Geneva. We waited, then, for the time to depart. On Sunday I heard Calvin preach to a large congregation, but I could not understand his sermon. I met one of my friends, Felix Irmi, who was studying French in Geneva.

We had to wait until the afternoon of the 17th of October for Monsieur Heroard. He came with a lackey and some brothers of Monsieur Potelière. We set out with them. We came before long to the bridge of Chancy, over the Rhône, and as night fell we entered Collonges, three leagues from Geneva. There we passed the night. Our horses were disturbed throughout the night because there was a mule in the stable, and I was obliged to get up to see to them. My horse had torn out the manger to which he had been fastened. I tied him up again elsewhere. I had not troubled to put on my shoes, and as a result my feet were frozen with cold. I had no sooner got back into bed than I was seized with such an upheaval of the belly that I had hardly time to get out again and to run out on to the gallery that encircled the inn. There I relieved myself of my torment. My companions, though sleeping in the same chamber, knew nothing of this. During the evening the surgeon had ordered his lackey to go in advance of us, early in the morning, to Nantua, to order a meal to be ready for us when we came there. When we got up, the innkeeper came to complain of the manner in which someone had used his gallery, and the wall below, which had been newly whitewashed. He declared that the front of his house was in an abominable state. The surgeon said that it must have been the lackey who was responsible for it, and persuaded the innkeeper that that was the reason why the man had left so early in the morning.

On the 18th of October, after leaving Collonges, we climbed a high mountain on the edge of the Rhône; there were several châteaux there. The river, in a deep gorge, fell over cataracts with a great roar. It is crossed by several bridges cut into the rock. We reached Châtillon, where there are cascades used to turn watermills. Beyond there we rode along a very bad road on the edge of a lake, which led us to Nantua, where we dined at the *Croix blanche*. Afterwards we went along the shore of a wild lake at the bottom of a narrow gorge. It was a dangerous road. Several times we saw the bodies of men hanging from the trees. The night came upon us as we descended the mountain, and it became so dark that we only just missed bumping into a corpse that was hanging from a branch. It made me shudder with fright. At last we came to Cerdon, three miles from Nantua, and there we lodged at the *Bois de Cerf.*

On the 19th we climbed a high mountain covered with chestnut trees and crowned by a fine château. Then we crossed a level plateau, to reach the little town of Saint-Maurice, where we descended at the *Chapeau de Cardinal.* After dinner we crossed the Ain[7] on a boat, and travelled afterwards across a plain to Montluel, where we lodged at the *Couronne,* a German hostelry whose master was quite drunk.

We arrived in Lyon on the 20th October, without having left the plain. As we came near the town we saw several men hanging from gibbets and others exposed on wheels. Schoepfius's horse started to limp, and he was obliged to do the rest of the journey to Lyon on foot. There we lodged at the *Ours,* which was kept by Paul Heberlin from Zurich. Everybody in the inn was German except the innkeeper. He had a stove in the room, a thing quite out of the ordinary in this country. Maître Heroardus went off to see people he knew in the town, and Schoepfius had to go and attend to his horse. He had bought it from Bernhardt Woelflin, of Basel, and had made a fool's bargain, for the beast, although of good appearance, had become ill and lame. He sold it later for next to nothing and had to go to Avignon by the Rhône.

I had to stay in Lyon the 21st and the 22nd, waiting for my companion from Montpellier, but in these two days I learned to appreciate the muscat of Montpellier. I went about the town, and having learned that Rondelet[8] was

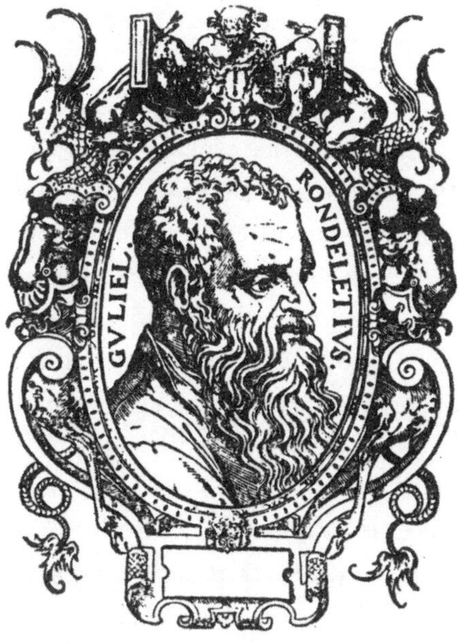

4. Rondelet, professor of the School of Medicine at Montpellier (from Rondelet, *Livre des Poissons*)

at Lyon with the Cardinal de Tournon, in the Saint-Jean quarter, I crossed the river to pay him a visit. There are always small boats, in charge of women, along the length of the quay, ready to transport you to the other shore. I took one of them and was thereby involved in a curious incident. In the middle of the river the woman demanded the fare. I had no change. She refused to put me ashore unless I paid her at once. We could not understand each other well, but she threatened to throw me into the water, or to take me lower down the river, which she began to do. To satisfy her I was obliged to give her a large pfennig, although I owed her no more than a sou, but she would not give me any change. When she put me ashore I threw stones at her. After this, Rondelet received me with the greatest good will. When I returned I went by way of the bridge to get to the inn, although that lengthened the journey. I learned also at Lyon that Colonel Schertlin, who had brought twenty companies to the king from Basel the preceding spring, had given battle to Colonel Martin Ross, and had gained a victory. I wrote this news to my father at the same time as I told him of our adventures on the way to Lyon; and that as we entered the town we had met a Christian[9] who was being led out to be burnt outside the gate; he was in his shirt with a truss of straw fastened on his back.

Early in the morning on the 23rd of October Thomas embarked on the Rhône. His departure made me very sad. After midday, Heroard, my companion, being ready, I left Lyon myself. We went by Saint-Symphorien to Vienne, a small and ancient town, where we stopped at the *Sainte-Barbe*. There we found Thomas again, with the boatmen and his fellow passengers. They had not been able to go any farther on account of contrary winds. So we passed the night together.

On the morning of the 24th of October we went outside the town to see an old pointed tower that the Romans had built in ancient times. It is a square pyramid, with an open base formed by the crossing of two arches, an extraordinary monument.

When we returned, Thomas embarked once more, while we remounted our horses. After about a mile we found ourselves once more by the Rhône, and we saw the boat coming down the river. We shouted greetings across the water to each other. A little farther on we came to a ford across a river, but the rain had swollen the stream so much that it was not prudent to attempt the crossing. We had been there only a moment when a great nobleman came, with five horses, who also wished to cross. It was the Master of the sons of King Henri,[10] who had come from court. He was very civil to us, and as the crossing was impossible he proposed that we should go to dine in the neighbourhood with a gentleman of his acquaintance, while we waited for the water to subside. He led us some distance from the road to a house, or rather to a farm, of poor appearance, where

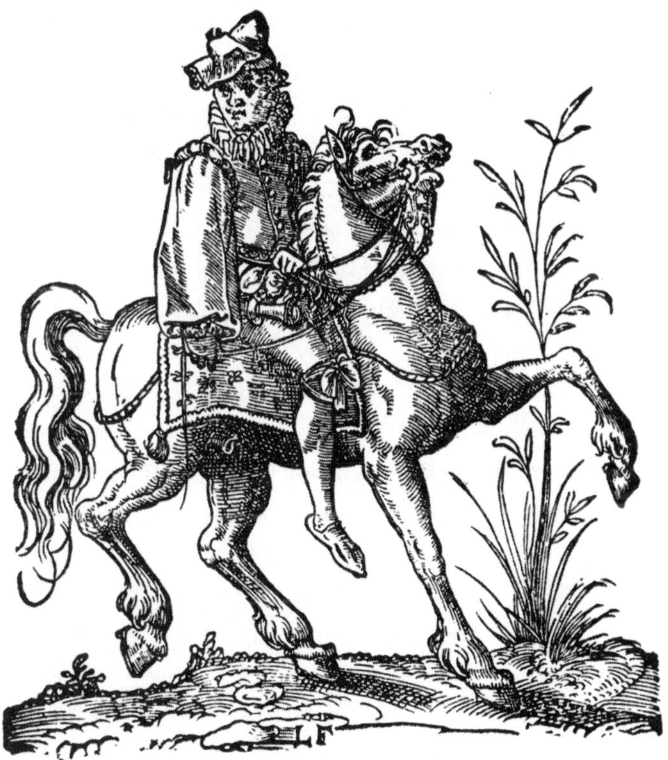

5. 'My little horse' (wood engraving by Jost Amman)

the gentleman in question, and his wife, made us very welcome. They gave us a sufficiently good meal, too, though none the less we had to pay for it. The nobleman who had brought us here talked with me in Latin, and asked for various information about Basel. I told him everything I knew about our laws and about our religion, and satisfied him. I pleased him so much that thereafter I had to ride constantly by his side and converse with him.

He sent one of his men to see if the level of the river had gone down. This man tried the ford on his horse, and returned to say that it was still very deep, but not impracticable. We got back into our saddles. I was apprehensive because of the small stature of my horse, but the nobleman took care to stay by my side, and gave me words of encouragement, and at last, thank God, I arrived safe and sound on the farther shore. My horse behaved valiantly on that occasion, as on all the rest of the journey.

By evening we arrived in the little town of Saint-Vallier, where we passed the night. The nobleman never tired of my conversation. His servants believed that they had to look after me at table, and each time that they brought me a glass, they would say '*Allons*', that is to say 'Come now'. I supposed that this word meant 'to drink' and each time that I wished for wine I would say to them '*Donnez-moi allons*'. They left me in this error for some time.

On the 25th we resumed our journey. We went towards a mountain where there was an ancient building called the House of Pilate. According to tradition Pontius Pilate came to live in the Dauphiné when he was exiled from Rome. Farther on, we came to the River Isère, which we had to cross on a ferry, and afterwards we entered Valence, where there is a university. We stayed at the *Dauphin*. After dinner the servant girl came to offer me a large pear, which she begged me to eat in her honour, but I was overcome by shyness and left without accepting it. After crossing the Drôme, also by ferry, we passed the little village of Livron, where the reformers afterwards put up so strong a resistance, and we spent the night at Loriol.

On the 26th of October, about midday, we reached the town of Montélimar, and by evening the market town of Pierrelatte, where I first saw olive-trees. They were heavy with fruit, some green, some red and half ripe, and some black and fully mature. I tried them all and found them nasty and very sour. By a road lined with olives we came on the 27th to the magnificent bridge of Saint-Esprit, by which we arrived at Orange. This is a small town, very ancient, and full of antiquities. We saw the Roman triumphal arch, which has some bas-reliefs on it, and also an old wall.[11] In the afternoon we were taken across a river and we entered Avignon. Monsieur the Master of the King's Children had taken leave of us some distance before this, to go farther into Provence, where he had a house, of which he told me the name, inviting me to come there to see him if I should ever make an excursion from Montpellier in the direction of Provence. On leaving us he had expressed his regard for me. When we reached Avignon, which is a considerable town belonging to the Pope, Michel Heroard left us to go to the house of a master minter of his acquaintance. He took me across to the other side of the Rhône to that quarter of Avignon called Villeneuve, to an inn called the *Coq*. It was a wretched shelter, where I found nothing but boatmen in wide breeches and blue caps.

They frightened me terribly because I was alone and with no one to talk to, and my fears prevented me from closing my eyes all night.

In the morning, the 28th of October, I rose very early. I was miserable and dejected, knowing no one, with no notion of how to find my travelling companion, and seeing around me none but coarse and rude people. I felt such a desire to return home that I went to the stable to my little horse and threw my arms round its neck and burst into tears. The poor beast, who was also alone, and whinnied plaintively for other horses, seemed to share the sorrow of our isolation. From there I went to a rock that overhangs the Rhône and gave myself up to sad thoughts. I felt myself abandoned by everyone. I blamed Maître Michel for going to Montpellier without me, and in my anger I tore up several pretty perfumed sachets that I had bought to send to my parents, and threw the pieces into the river. But God came to my assistance. I went into a church. It was Sunday, and the sound of the organ, together with the singing, calmed my temper a little. I returned to the inn, and after a lonely meal, not knowing what to do, I threw myself on my bed, and, quite against my custom, fell into a sound slumber. When evening came I went to Vespers, in order to hear a little music, and sat glumly down in a corner; but on my returning to the inn, there was Maître Michel's lackey, who had come to tell me to be ready early in the morning. I bade him to tell his master that I could not spend another night in the inn, because the boatmen would surely murder me. Michel sent for me and brought me to supper in the house of his friend the minter, who gave me a bed in his house, in a chamber in which there were several balances with bronze money, which was afterwards declared false and forbidden. I recovered my spirits.

In the morning, the 29th, I recrossed the Rhône to return to the inn. The innkeeper wrote on a board, with chalk, the sum I owed him, all the time reciting his Pater Noster in Latin. I was obliged to give him all that he demanded, for I understood nothing of his speech.

As I saddled my horse, Michel came, and we departed. At the first hill my horse began to limp badly, and this terrified me because I was afraid that I should be left on the road; but when I examined his hoof I saw that the cause was only a stone that had lodged under the shoe. I pulled it out and the beast recovered its usual pace.

We crossed the River Gard on a ferry, and arrived towards midday at Sernhac, where we dined at the *Angel*. The innkeeper's daughter tried to kiss me, but I would not have it, which caused a lot of laughter, for it is the custom in this country to welcome with a kiss. At night we entered Nîmes, where we lodged at the *Pomme rouge*.

Early in the morning I went out to see the antiquities of Nîmes. In the great amphitheatre there is a group of Romulus and Remus suckled by a she-wolf, and another statue of a man standing erect, with three faces.

From Nîmes the road crossed a plain set with olive-trees as far as Lunel, where I drank the first wine of the muscat. After dinner we rested on our beds for a short time, because the heat was heavy at that time of the year, when in our country it is still midwinter. Maître Michel was delighted that he was coming near his home, and I too was happy to know that we should be in Montpellier before evening. We travelled on to Chambéry, the town to which the Germans of Montpellier accompany any of their number leaving for home. Not far from there we came to a hill with a cross on it, and from there for the first time we saw Montpellier and the sea. A little farther on we crossed the bridge near the inn at Castelnau, and afterwards passed the place of execution,[12] which is in the fields in front of the town. Pieces of human flesh hung from the olive trees, and this sight gave me a curious sensation. At last, by the grace of God, we entered the gates of Montpellier early on a Sunday evening. I prayed then to God to give me grace to complete my studies in this town, and to bring me safe and sound back to my own country and to my family.

On entering we met a large number of the inhabitants, of the nobility and others, clothed in long white shirts, and walking about the streets, preceded by stringed instruments and banners. They carried in their hands shells of silver full of sugared almonds,[13] and struck upon them

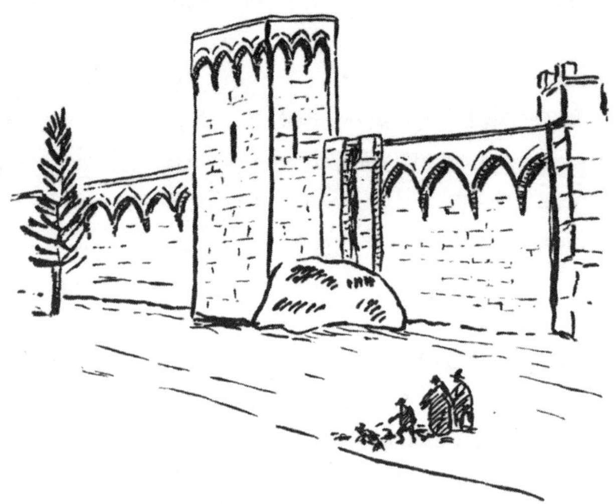

6. The walls of Montpellier (drawing by Seán Jennett)

with spoons of the same metal, and offered their sweets to every pretty girl they found in their path. This spectacle dissipated my sombre thoughts. Maître Michel showed me the house of Laurent Catalan, at the corner of the square, and then left me to go to his own house.

Monsieur Laurent and his wife Eléonore were watching the diversion going on in front of their shop,[14] which, as was customary, was closed on Sundays. They were surprised when they saw me dismount. I addressed him in Latin and gave him the letter from Doctor Volffius, his son's former tutor. He gave a sigh, and then ordered that my horse should be taken to his brother-in-law's stable.

Soon after Johann Odratzheim arrived. He was a Strasbourger and served in the pharmacy. He bade me welcome and took me into the house. The servant Beatrice took off my boots. She was hanged later, as I shall describe.

My journey from Basel to Montpellier had taken twenty days, from the 10th to the 30th of October; but we had really been no more than fifteen days travelling, and during that time we had covered ninety-five miles.[15] My expenses had amounted to 10 *livres* 12 *schellings*, and 10 *deniers*, including fodder and stabling for the horse, tips, and tolls across rivers.

2

A STUDENT IN MONTPELLIER

Monsieur Catalan told me at once that Jacob Meier, of Strasbourg, who had lived in his house as an exchange for his son Jacques, had died of a *febre continuâ*. He was very distressed, and feared too that his son Jacques, who was in Strasbourg with the dead boy's father, might now be less well treated, and might even be obliged to pay for his keep. I conceived at once the hope of persuading Catalan to send his son to my father's house in Basel, as an exchange for me. I could thus enjoy the benefit of an exchange, and Monsieur Catalan would keep me with him all the more willingly while he settled the question of his two sons, both in Strasbourg—for soon Johann Odratzheim would also be returning home. So now I had a double opportunity for an exchange.

I found several Germans in Montpellier: Jacob Baldenberg, of Saint-Gall, who had begun his studies in Basel; Petrus Lotichius, the distinguished poet, who was a tutor with the Stibare family, relations of the Bishop of Würzburg; George Stetus, from Leipzig; and Johann Vogelsang, a

Flammand. They had all been several years in Montpellier. I also found Thomas Schoepfius there, for he had arrived before me.

I was not long in acclimatizing myself. The weather was still very hot, and the harvest of the olives had only just begun. Peasants are employed for this work and they knock the fruit down with long poles. They gathered in a crowd early one morning, in front of our shop, making a great noise. The tumult roused me, and when I looked out between the shutters I thought that the square was full of armed men with lances. This frightened me, but Odratzheim told me that they were only labourers.

I began without delay to follow the curriculum of the school. I also wrote to my father that Jacob Meier was dead and that there was a chance that one or other of the Catalan sons would be sent to his house—their father had given me his word on it. I told him about our adventures on the way, and added some details about Montpellier. For example, large numbers of Bibles and other religious books that our people had had printed and which had been found at a bookseller's, had been burned publicly in the street. Finally, that my master had given me eight crowns for my horse, and with that money I had bought a *flassada*, made of Catalan cloth,[16] to keep me warm at night, and several other garments.

On the 4th of November I was examined by Doctor Honoré Castellan, and as a result I was matriculated, and was informed so in writing by Doctor Guichard. Later, when I was admitted to study for a baccalaureate, I was sent a printed card: *Descriptus fuit in albo studiosorum medicinae M. Felix Platerus, per manus, anno Domini 1552, die vero*

4 novembris; cujus pater est venerandus D. Saporta, nostrae Academiae decanus, qui ejusdem jura persolvit. Datum Monspessuli ut supra. P. Guichard. (Felix Platter has been inscribed by our hands in the book of students of medicine in the year I 552, the 4th of November. His sponsor is Doctor Saporta, dean of our Academy, who has accepted this obligation. Given at Montpellier, as hereunder. Doctor Guichard.)

I had chosen Doctor Saporta as my sponsor, for it is the custom for each student to choose one, so that he may have someone whom he may consult. It was Catalan who sent me to Doctor Saporta, to whom I had also been recommended from another quarter.

On the 6th of November I went to Villeneuve, in company with a number of Germans. I was very surprised to see rosemary growing in the fields as freely as the juniper does with us. There were marjoram and thyme as well, filling the fields, and so common that no one pays any attention to them. Rosemary is used for heating, there is so much of it. It is carried into the town on the backs of donkeys, and burned in the hearths. A load under which an ass can scarcely be seen costs not more than a *carolus*, which is equal to a double piece of four. For cooking they burn logs of a wood called ilex. It is a kind of oak; its berries give a scarlet dye, or cramoisy. The last name comes from the berry, which is called *kermès*; it contains little worms, which give the tincture, and if the berries are not gathered in time, the worms grow wings and fly out of the shell.

I made arrangements for a course of serious study. I would attend two or three lectures in the morning, and as many more in the afternoon. From the 14th a dissection was conducted in the old theatre on the corpse of a boy who had died of an abscess in the stomach *(pleuritide)*. Inside his chest, *in succingente membranâ*, there was only a blue stain with neither swelling nor abscess. The lung was attached by ligaments that had to be cut before it could be taken out. Doctor Guichard presided at this autopsy, and a barber did the operation. Besides the students, the audience contained many people of the nobility and the bourgeoisie, and even young girls, notwithstanding that the subject was a male. There were even some monks present.

On the 4th of December we went to see the sources of the Lez,[17] which is called Ledum in Latin. It rises half a day's journey from Montpellier, in the Gerus, and falls over a cascade; it flows to Castelnau, very near Montpellier, and joins the sea not far from that town. Its whole length, from its source to the sea, is no more than a day's walk. At the source, under the cascade, there are stones as round as marbles.

The month of December was seldom cold, and we saw neither ice nor snow such as we have at home. To warm themselves the students keep a fire of rosemary burning, and it gives a good flame and a sweet smell. Bedrooms are kept well closed, but the windows are only frames covered with paper in place of glass.

A great procession was held, with many priests and monks. The monstrance, with the sacrament, was carried through the streets. It was a supplication for the benefit of the King of France, that he might come safely out of the war against Charles V. The latter was then besieging Metz, which the king had won from the empire.

Doctor Jacob Hugguelin, who had studied medicine in Basel, arrived on the 28th of December. He brought me news of my father, and a letter dated the 27th of November. My father told me that Basel was in great danger because of the war with Charles V. Troops filled the country from Strasbourg to Metz, and were besieging the latter town, despite the rigours of winter. He added that mortality from the plague was still great in Basel, and that want was now added to it. He enjoined me to behave well, so that I might remain with my master. He had written to me previously, but I had not yet received that letter, and it did not reach me until later, as I shall describe.

On Christmas eve the merchants' shops were full of coloured candles, which the people buy and light on this night. The two assistant apothecaries, and also Johann Odratzheim, who shared my bed with me, went off to midnight mass, as the custom was when the town was still papist. I found myself alone in the great house, and I was very frightened. I took a lamp and shut myself in the study, which was at the top of the house, and was a plain little closet lined with boards. I stayed there until they returned from mass, reading the comedy of *Amphitryon* in an old copy of Plautus.

The new year brought all sorts of amusements, and in particular serenades, sung by gallants under the windows of the houses. The instruments they played included cymbals, a drum, and a fife, the same musician playing all three instruments at once; the hautboy, which was very common, the viol, and a guitar, which was then a novelty. The rich bourgeois give balls, to which young ladies may be taken. After supper, in the light of torches, they dance the *branle*, the *gaillard*, the *volte*, the *tire-chaîne*, and others, and go on until the morning. These balls continue until the last day of the festivities.

One day I went to fetch Doctor Griffy's daughter, to bring her to a ball, as the custom was. While walking with her past a midden, and wishing to give her the best side of the street, unhappily I put my foot in the mud and splashed her from head to foot with that filthy water. I was quite confused, and dismayed when a friend who was with us went ahead and announced that I had offered holy water to my fiancée. The young lady saw at once that I had no malicious intention and begged me to take her back home to change her garments, which I did.

During the early days of January a procession was held, with public prayers that the king should be victorious. We Germans celebrated the Feast of the Kings[18] with a superb banquet and a concert, at which I played the lute. At that time the fields were so covered with a kind of hyacinth as to appear all blue.

On the 12th of January I received from my father a letter dated the 13th of November. It had been sent by means of some merchants going to Lyon, and had suffered a long delay, for its date was earlier than that of the letter brought to me by Hugguelin. It was the first that my father had sent to me at Montpellier. He told me that his servant Anna Oswald had caught the plague, and had fortunately recovered from it. He had sent away all his boarders because of the mortality, which was still severe. The French ambassador Morelet had died on the 17th of October; he used to live in Basel in a house that now belongs to Lux Iselin, and was formerly called the Hôtel de France. He closed his letter by enjoining me to fear God and to work hard, and told me to stay with Catalan, so that he might take Gilbert Catalan in exchange, from Strasbourg, as soon as the plague had ceased; for it would be quite impossible for him to furnish me with money to live abroad.

My father's letter redoubled my desire to learn, and this pleased old Catalan. He loved to talk to me in Latin, and when I replied in Latin better than his, he would marvel.

After supper, when we were warming ourselves by the hearth, Monsieur Catalan[19] gave me an old Latin Bible, from which the New Testament was missing. I read it to him, and commented upon it. When I read the prophet Baruch, who preaches against images and idols, Catalan was delighted. He was a Maran,[20] and loved idols no more than do the Jews; but he did not dare to declare so openly. He interrupted me often with the words '*Ergo nostri sacerdotes*', that is to say, Why do our priests have them? I replied that the priests were wrong, and that our religion rejected such images and idols, and I cited a host of passages in which God had forbidden them. This pleased him, and he asked how I could know so many things at my age. He took me for a well of knowledge. I explained to him that my father was a *gymnasiarque*, or the head of a school, and that it was he who had taught me, at the same time as he had taught his students. This confirmed Catalan in his decision to send his son Gilbert from Strasbourg to my father as soon as possible. He wrote to Gilbert then to go Basel at the first opportunity, and I was very pleased that I should thus have contributed some part to ensure a good exchange. All the same, some doubts remained with me because of the plague that still raged in Basel, and of which

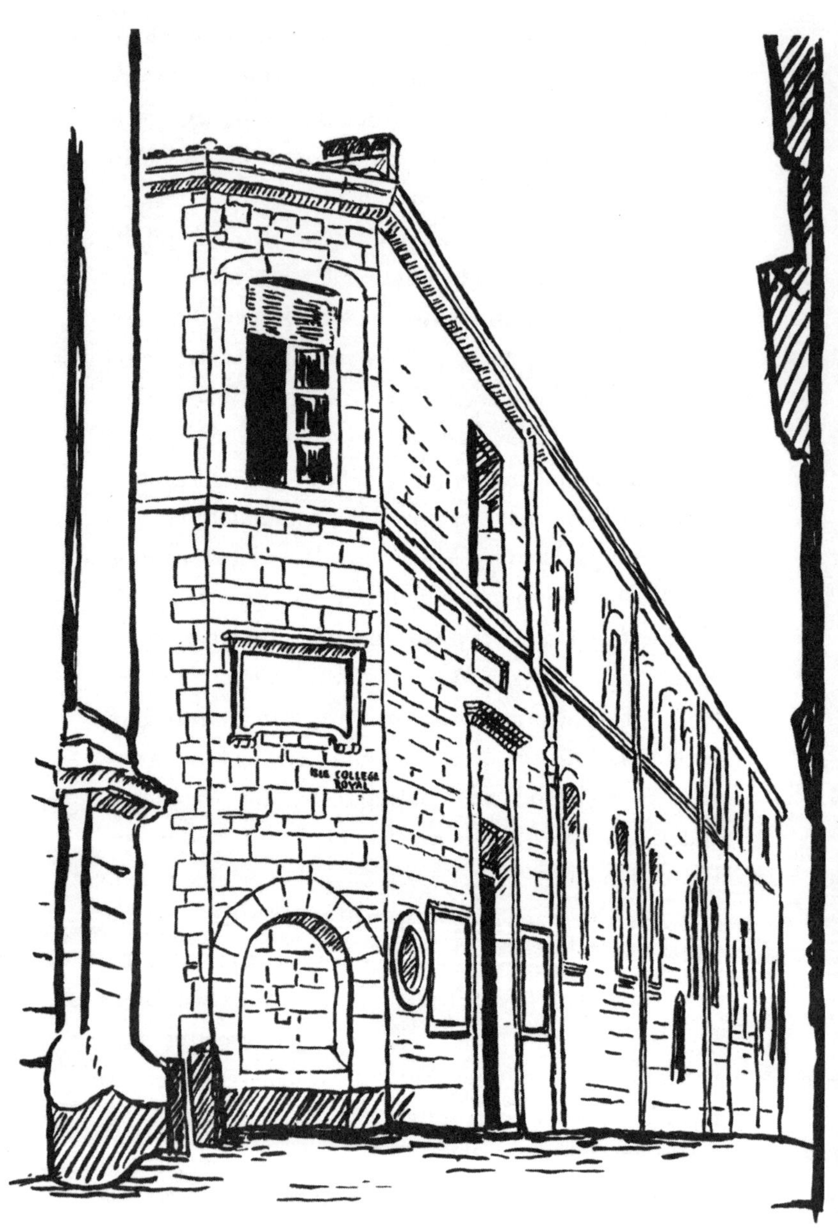

7. The College today (drawing by Seán Jennett)

my master knew nothing. I had hidden this fact from him, because if I had not he would have refused to receive me when I first arrived, as coming from an infected town.

On the 14th of January I wrote again to my father, and explained to him the advantages that Montpellier offered for the study of medicine, on account of the teaching there, the anatomy sessions, and so forth. I had in addition the advantage of my master's shop, which was large and employed four or five assistants. There I saw something new every day. My master and his wife loved me as their own son. Among political news, I told him that the King of France had just concluded a treaty with the Turks. Catalan also wrote to my father, and said that it was his intention to give his son Gilbert into his care, and to send his other son Jacques to the house of the secretary of Basel, whose son Frederick, then in Paris, proposed to return to Montpellier. I wrote also to my mother, as well as to Johann Huber, Peter Gebwiler, *greffier* of Roetelen, in whose house I had stayed, my cousin Laurenz Offner, then in Strasbourg, and to my friends Martin Hubert and Daniel Vieland.

On the 8th of February a number of Germans left Montpellier to return home to Würzburg by way of Basel. They were Erhardus and Martinus Stibare, kinsmen of the Bishop of Würzburg, Georgius Fischerus, their tutor, and Locherus. We accompanied them as far as the village of Saint-Brès, where we passed the night joyously in all kinds of follies.

I took the opportunity of their going to write a letter to my father, to whom my master also wrote to say that as soon as the plague had left Basel he should receive Gilbert Catalan and take him *en pension*, while the *greffier* of Basel would take his son Jacques, provided that Frederic Rihener wrote from Paris that he would not further delay his return to Montpellier.

On the 12th of February, the day that is called Shrove Sunday in our calendar, there were further serenades and masquerades of all sorts in Montpellier. They went on all day on Monday and all day on Tuesday, which is called Mardi Gras here. On this day young people roved through the town with bags full of oranges hung round their necks. This fruit is sold ridiculously cheap in this country, and a dozen of them cost no more than a *patart*, that is to say, two *deniers*.[21] These people also carry baskets, which they use as shields. They gathered in the Place Notre-Dame and hurled the oranges against each other, and soon the whole square was strewn with debris.

Lent commences with Ash Wednesday. Meat and eggs are forbidden under pain of death, but we Germans did not stop eating them. I learned how to cook eggs in butter on a piece of paper held over live charcoal. I did not dare to use any utensil for this purpose. Throughout Lent I collected in my study the shells of eggs that I had cooked there, in this manner, over the flame of a candle, but a servant discovered them and showed them to my mistress, who was very annoyed. However, she did not take the matter further.

It is the custom to break all earthenware vessels that have been used for meat, and to buy new ones in Lent for fish.

We lived frugally in my master's house. The cooking was done in Spanish fashion, although the Marans abstain from the same foods as do the Jews. At midday we eat a soup garnished with *naveaux*[22] or cabbage; it contains mutton, rarely beef, and is not in plenty. It is eaten with the fingers, each person from his own dish. At supper salad is served regularly, and is followed by a small roast; the remains of this would not give anyone indigestion. Bread is in sufficient quantity, and is very good. There is wine for those who want it; it is deep red in colour, and is drunk mixed with water, The servant first pours as much water as you wish, and then adds the wine. If you do not drink all of it, what is left is thrown away. This wine does not keep more than a year, and turns sour.

We had a more scanty fare during Lent. First, we would have a soup made with cabbage prepared with oil; then would follow haddock, a kind of fish that resembles cod. We had other sea fish too, for example small soles, seasoned with oil and cooked on a stove while we were at the table, and served on a little plate. Sometimes we had tunny, a kind of fish four or five feet long. Cooking is always done with oil, and I did not eat anything cooked in butter during the whole of my stay in Montpellier. There are also mackerel and sardines, which are very good boiled or fried; eels, which are abundant; enormous lobsters *(langustae)* two feet long, and small lobsters without pincers *(squillae)*, which are brought in in basketsful. Unfortunately, they were not often seen in our house. At supper time, even in Lent, we had a salad of lettuce or blanched chicory, and sometimes some onions. Onions are sold in the market in great heaps about the time of Saint Bartholomew's day. They are cooked in syrup. During most of the winter we also had roasted chestnuts, but never cheese or fruit.

The fine weather and the heat returned with the month of February. I was impatient to see the sea, which so far I had only viewed from a distance; so on the 22nd of

February we went to the village of Pérols, which is on the edge of a lagoon and about two leagues from Montpellier. In a meadow near the village we saw a pit in which water bubbled noisily, as though it were boiling, though none the less it was as cold as ice. They say that the king once made one of his lackeys drink some of the water, and that the man died on the spot.

We came to the shore of the salt lagoon, which is long, but so shallow that one could almost ford it. There was a boat there, but without oars and with no one to steer it. We had no other recourse than to haul it to the other side by the rope, and some of us sat in it while the others pulled.[23] In this way we came to the strip of land that divided the

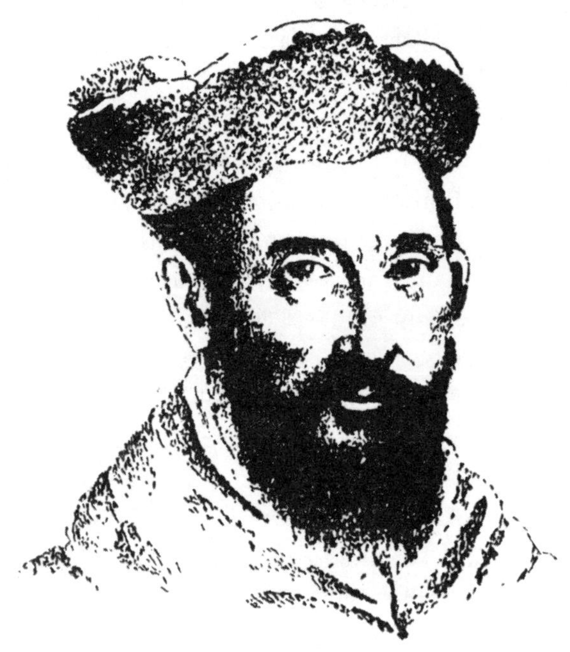

8. Schyron, professor of the School of Medicine at Montpellier

lagoon from the sea, and which is in many places no more than twenty paces across, though solid enough to defy both wave and tempest. There is an abundance of maritime plants, and the beach is covered with so many shells and cuttlefish bones that one might fill a wagon with them. As the waves withdraw they uncover stretches of sand, but they return almost at once, and if you are not quick enough, then you have your shoes and stockings filled up with water. We undressed and bathed. It was not yet Saint Matthew's day, but the water was already pleasant, and the sand on the beach was so warm that when we came out of the sea we covered ourselves with it to take off the chill of the water. It is an excellent means of firming the skin, and of curing the ringworm. I gathered a number of shells of all colours, some crabs, and many other curiosities. The crabs are abundant, and are round and run sideways. We recrossed the lagoon for a meal at Pérols, and then we returned to Montpellier.

The lectures were numerous. In the morning there were those of Sabranus, Saporta, and Schyronius, and at nine o'clock that of Rondelet.[24] In the afternoon there were those of Fontanonus, Bocaudus, Guichardus, and Griffius. We breakfasted during Schyronius's period, for he was very old, and one day he filled his breeches in his professorial chair. We would pass an hour in the *Trois Rois*, in the faubourg, not far from the College,[25] where we would get a measure of excellent muscat for a *stüler*, that is to say a *batzen* or a *carolus*, which is equal to a piece of four. With this we might have meat—some pork, for example, with a little mustard—for we never had this in my master's house. The cost was less than a *stüber* for each of us. In March in this year a large number of students were made bachelors. Among them was a Spaniard, who had obtained special permission to stay here, for at that time Spaniards were not allowed to come to study in Montpellier. Among the bachelors there was one Galorius, who had studied at Basel and had been an exchange there for Tigurinus Schneeberger. He often frequented people of our nation, and later became a doctor in Kraków in Poland. About the same time Monsieur Fischerus was also promoted to the degree of licentiate, in a magnificent ceremony that took place in the courtyard of the bishop's house.

Georg Fischerus, the Stibares' tutor, who had accompanied his pupils on their journey as far as Lyon, returned to Montpellier on the 9th of March, and Michael Hoffmann arrived from Hall on the 2nd of April.

On the 6th of April my books arrived from Basel. Monsieur Gabriel Fry had sent them to Lyon for me, and Monsieur Thomas Guérin, a bookseller of that town, had sent them on to Montpellier by means of Bonhomme, a printer, also of Lyon.

We went to Villeneuve on the 7th of April, with the intention of visiting Maguelone, which lies between the lagoon and the sea. We could not find a boat to cross the lagoon, and we had to return to Montpellier.

On the 22nd Catalan's wife was brought to bed of a child. Her name had been Eléonore Biersch, and she was the daughter of Raphael Biersch. She had several brothers who were traders, and a sister in Lyon, married to a Spanish doctor, Jean de la Sala. All the family were Marans. She gave birth to the child in the dining room, behind a curtain, and brought forth a son. He was called Laurent, and was secretly circumcized and baptized according to their custom.

On the 2nd of May I received a letter from Frederick Rihener. He was undecided whether to come to Montpellier or to go to Italy.

On the 5th of May, Thomas Schoepfius, who had come with me from Basel to Montpellier, returned home to his wife and children. On the way he took his doctorate at Valence. I gave him a letter to take to my father. In it I explained how it was that Catalan's son had not yet joined him in Basel, despite the promise made in February. The reason was that Conrad Forer, of Winterthür, who was nicknamed the Babbler, because he was always talking out of turn, had told Catalan that the plague was raging in Basel, and had declared himself surprised that he should propose to send his son there at such a time. Monsieur Catalan reproached me for having concealed the fact. He was in an ill humour, brought on by a disagreement he had had with one of his former boarders, Henry Rihener, the son of the secretary of Basel, who became a doctor, married, and settled down at Salers, in Auvergne. He still owed money to Catalan, whom he had told to send to his father for it: but the elder Rihener had referred Catalan back to the son, under the pretence that the son had acted against his father's wishes. This double annoyance caused Catalan to change his mind, and now he no longer wanted to send his son Jacques to the secretary in Basel, nor Gilbert to my father's house. He had therefore approached a merchant of Lyon, who would pass through Strasbourg as he returned from the fair at Frankfurt, and asked him to bring both sons back with him to Lyon, from which town they would return to Montpellier. We heard soon afterwards that they were on their way. This news frightened me, and I went to the pharmacy in company with Schoepfius, who took my part, and asked Catalan if there was any truth in the rumours that were spread about. He affirmed that they were correct, and complained bitterly about Henry. But he had no complaint to make about me—he liked me very much, and would not have me embarrassed or disturbed. I explained that it was not possible for my father to pay for my keep while I was in Montpellier, and I reminded him that he had given me some reason to hope for an exchange. I passed that day sad and dispirited. At supper Catalan noticed my low spirits and said that he would have great pleasure in sending his son to my father, and that he was ashamed of having decided otherwise: and that if his sons were still in Lyon he would send them word by Thomas Schoepfius, who was then about to leave, that Jacques, the younger of the two, should go to my father's house, while the elder returned to Montpellier. Moreover, if these counter-orders should arrive too late, then he would take me as tutor to one of his children as the price of my lodging, a practice common among the students.

As it happened, the merchants of Montpellier returned from Lyon before Schoepfius left, about Easter, and without the two Catalan sons. The merchant of Lyon, who had been to Frankfurt and should have brought them back to Lyon, had not passed by way of Strasbourg. My joy was unbounded when my master gave me this news. I told my father at once, by a letter that I gave to Thomas, that he should take Jacques Catalan into his house as soon as the plague was ended, and send Gilbert to Lyon. I took this opportunity to ask him to send me a folio copy of the works of Galen.

On the 8th of May Monsieur Salomon,[26] also called Monsieur d'Assas, whose mother had several German boarders in her house, was promoted licentiate with great solemnity, and according to custom.

My master had a house and lands in a village called Vendargues. The bailiff of this property was one Gillem, who had taken the two Catalan boys to Basel in the panniers of an ass. He had been converted to our religion, and often spoke against the papists, especially when he had had too much to drink, which was often since he had been to Germany. Indeed, I never saw anyone drunk in Montpellier other than Germans. I went on horseback to the property, in company with my master's brother-in-law. Each one of us took a Maran girl on the croup. We stayed the night there. At this place I saw goats with long, flapping ears. These animals are common in this country, and are called *cabri*. I also saw a number of peacocks[27] from the Indies; they are fed entirely on grass, and are driven in great herds to market.

At Pentecost I put on new breeches that were red in colour. They were tight, slashed, and lined with taffeta, and pleated so low that I almost sat on the gathers. They were so tight that I could scarcely bend. They cost me no more than a crown, however, and the crown was then worth forty-six *stübers*. The tailors themselves supply the material, and in case of need will make you a pair of breeches between the evening and the morning.

As early as Shepherd's Day we were eating ripe cherries. These are sold by the pound, as also are the figs called *grossos*, which are enormous. These are the first figs, for this tree produces two crops. The second, which ripens in the autumn, is the better.

On the 23rd of May I went for a walk outside the gates of the town. I gathered some pomegranate blossoms—there are many of these trees in the district—and took them back with me. As I came into the Place Notre-Dame, which is used as a promenade, I saw two German students who had just arrived. I recognized them at once, for they were from Basel. One was Jacob Geischüsler, who was called Myconius, because he was the adoptive son of Oswald Myconius. The other was Balthazar Hummel, who had been an assistant to Thomas, the apothecary, where my father had placed him when he had left his school. They had come as far as Lyon, from Basel, in the company of Zacharie, the son of Gladius, the innkeeper of the *Wild Man*.

On the same day five martyrs were burned, who had studied at Lausanne, and who on their return had been arrested, thrown into prison, and condemned to the fire. Myconius and Hummel watched their execution. They recounted all the details, which have been put down in the Book of Martyrs. Myconius had recently received a small bequest from Oswald, but not a sou remained when he returned to Basel. Hummel had been given three crowns and a horse by his father. He had sold the horse on the way for three more crowns, and now all was spent. His father, a professional soldier, had also given him a cloak, which originally had been white and black, but had been dyed black all over; the former pattern could be seen once more under the dye.

They brought me a letter, dated the 7th of April, in which my father gave me all kinds of news. Margarethe, a relative of my mother's, who had been brought up with us, had been claimed and taken away by her father, Germain Dietschin. Her departure had made my parents very sad. Captain Irmi Nicolas was dead; he had been brought back very ill from Paris, and I learned later that he had had a shameful disease. The plague had gone from Basel, and my father had found new boarders. The question of Catalan's sons was settled. Oporinus would bring them with him when he returned from Frankfurt. The secretary of Basel understood that my father would take them both until such time as Frederick should return to Montpellier, when he would himself take Jacques. My father had borrowed ten crowns from the secretary to bring the two boys from Strasbourg to Basel; this amount was what one Isaac Cellarius owed to Catalan. He also told me how ungrateful Myconius had shown himself to be, and counselled me not to allow myself to be led astray by him or by Hummel, but to continue with my work. He said that the town beadle had been found guilty of embezzling the pay of the *lansquenets*, and had been put in prison; he was later exiled to Vienna, in Austria, where he became a halberdier.

This letter had been written since the 7th of April, but for want of a messenger it did not leave until the 3rd of May. My father had added a postscript on the 12th of April, announcing with despair that the two Catalan sons had arrived at his house with the news that their father had recalled them to Montpellier. He thought that it must be because Monsieur Catalan had found some reason to complain of my conduct, to have changed his mind so quickly. Moreover, Gilbert did not want to leave, believing that his father had recalled him only because he was afraid that he might become a protestant, and he was therefore going to write to suggest that only the younger brother Jacques should be recalled, while he himself remained in Basel. There he would have much to learn from my father. In any case, there seemed now to be little likelihood that Frederick would return from Paris to Montpellier, for his father had died on the 18th of April, carried off by some disease of the head, as also were his two stewards, and his loss was mourned by all the town. I must, then, beg my master to agree to the exchange of Gilbert for me, and my father himself asked for this in a letter brought by the same messenger. I was appalled. I must once more explain to my father how my master had altered his mind, and exculpate myself. Eight days later I found the occasion to send a letter.

On the 29th of May Georg Stet, of Leipzig, quitted Montpellier, and I took advantage of his going to write to my father. I told him that my master had changed his mind, Jacques was to have remained in Basel, while Gibert returned to Montpellier. I feared that Gilbert might be already on the way; for now Monsieur Catalan had decided, that very evening, to leave him too in Basel, and to pay my father for Jacques's keep. There, I said, see what I have succeeded in arranging—I was far from being out of favour with my master. As it was, I should not only enjoy the benefit of an exchange, but I should have money to clothe me out of what Catalan should pay for Jacques.

Myconius seized upon this first opportunity to accompany Germans on their way home. We went with them as far as Frontignan, the country of the muscat. He sat at table there, with others, in Salomon's house, and feasted in high style. His medical studies were now well advanced. Hummel wanted to go to Piedmont, to a posting house kept by Baptista there, who had lodged with his master Thomas and had given him a marvellous account of the country; but he had no money and was quite cast down. Seeing this, I interceded with my master to take him into his pharmacy in place of Odratzheim, who was due to leave for Toulouse in four days' time. At first Catalan raised objections because Hummel knew no French, but he consented in the end, on condition that Hummel should receive no wages the first year. Hummel would have to make do with tips, which he would share with two or three other assistants.

My master now declared that he would definitely leave his two sons with my father, for the elder begged to be left in Basel, so that his studies should not be further interrupted. They would stay there two or three years, and perhaps longer, under the conditions now agreed: one should be an exchange for me, and the other should be paid for, the money to be put into my hands to maintain my wardrobe. I was given some of this money immediately, so that I might have a Spanish cap made for me, and buy a lute, which proved to be excellent and cost only three francs. Thus was my future assured, as far as my doctorate at least. I gave thanks to God, marvelling at the ways of Providence, which had made Gilbert, as he passed through Geneva, on his way to Lyon, meet a pretty young girl and no longer wish to leave. He had at once taken to writing letter after letter to his father, asking to be allowed to stay in Basel for the furtherance of his studies, but the real reason was that he wanted to court the girl, and by letters and presents persuade her to marry him. In the end Gilbert turned out a man of poor account, frequenting the card table more than the study, and he became a philanderer and malicious.

My master decided to move his pharmacy from the corner of the square, where it had been, to his own house on the corner opposite. I had to move my lodging to another of his houses, a veritable palace, which he had inherited from a Doctor Falcon,[28] a Spaniard and a Maran also. At first I was given a vast chamber, but afterwards I installed myself in a little boarded study on the upper floor. I decorated it with my pictures, and my master put in a gilded armchair—for he showed me all sorts of kindness now that his two sons were with my father. At the top of the house there was a fine terrace, or platform,[29] reached by a stone stair. It commanded the whole town, and one could see as far as the sea, the sound of which could be heard when the wind was in the right quarter. This was where I liked to study. I grew an Indian fig tree there in a vase—my master had been sent a leaf of it from Spain.

I was alone in the house, and took my meals in the pharmacy, which was not far away, but in the evening Hummel would return with me, and share my bed, so that I might not be alone during the night. As he loved the lute, I would sit at the window and play it, and the people in the house opposite, which belonged to Monsieur de Saint-Georges, would come and listen, especially his sister, Mistress Marthe Guichard de Sandre.

On the 26th of June Stephen Contzenus left Montpellier for Strasbourg, where his fiancée was, and I sent a letter by him to my father, to tell him that the Catalan sons were

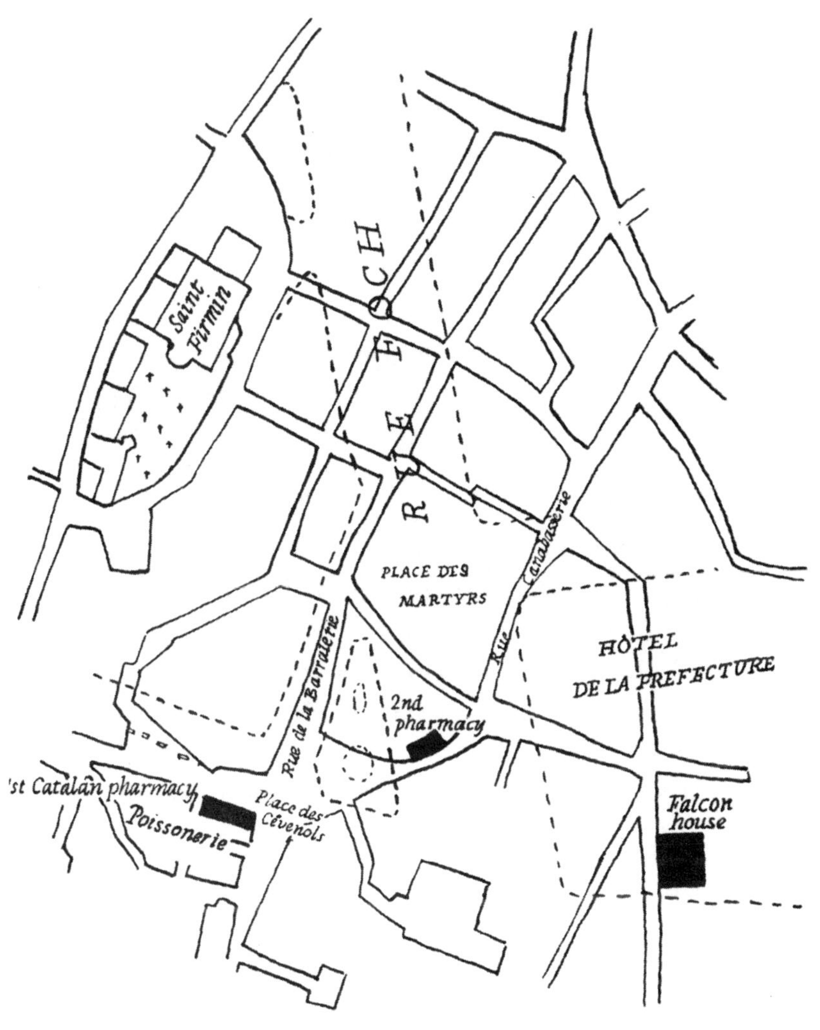

9. Plan of the centre of Montpellier, showing the site of the two Catalan pharmacies and the house of Dr. Falcon. The position of the present Rue Foch is shown dotted. Modern place names are in capitals (drawing by Seán Jennett)

to remain in his house. My master also wrote to confirm this good news, and sent an acknowledgement for the ten crowns that were owed to him by Isaac Cellarius; my father was to collect this money to repay the ten crowns he had borrowed from the secretary. Monsieur Catalan also asked if my father would do what he could to collect the money owed to him by Henry Rihener as soon as that gentleman got possession of his paternal heritage.

On the 22nd of July a baker's son was executed. He was a fine young man. He was taken to the Place Notre-Dame, near the church, where a scaffold had been built of planks, with a block supported on a beam. The executioner bandaged the young man's eyes, and then laid him down on his stomach, with his neck bare across the block. He then drew out a great sword, which he had kept hidden beneath his cloak, and struck the condemned man two blows on the neck. The severed head rolled across the floor. Afterwards the executioner cut off both legs and both arms, and arranged them on the scaffold with the head in the middle, and left them there all night. In the morning he hung them on an olive-tree outside the town and there they were left to rot.

On the 25th of July we went to Gramont to collect plants. It is a little monastery, not far from the town, and in the middle of a copse of oaks (*ilices*) and *cisti ledi*, etc. There were many wild rabbits there, but no one is allowed to take them, except the monks of the monastery, who are both few and poor. Against the wall of the monastery is a roofed tomb, bearing a sculptured shield charged with two keys. It is said that this is the tomb of the knight Peter,

Count of Provence, who freed Maguelone from the rule of Naples, as is recorded in the history of Maguelone.

Next to the house in which I lodged lived a doctor of law, whose wife and cousin often came to sit on the roof, with their needlework, to hear me play the lute.

On the 1st of August Jacob Baldenbergius left for Toulouse. He later became a doctor at Saint-Gall. He was a great Hellenist, but was as debauched as he was learned.

On the 3rd of August I wrote home. I spoke of the excessive heat of the dog days, from which one could get relief only by watering the floors, and by hanging sheets and branches in the streets to give shade.[30] There had been no rain now for a long time.

On the 10th of August, Saint Lawrence's day, my master took me to see his vine. On leaving he had said to Balthazar Hummel, '*Bautasach, accipe tuum gladium*', thinking that he would bring a knife to cut the grapes; but what Hummel came out with was a sword. Then my master said: '*Vis pugnare?*' ('Do you want a battle?'), and told him that by the word *gladius* he had intended a knife.

The vine was extensive, and loaded down with large black grapes—white grapes are seldom grown, other than the muscat, which is golden and exquisite. There is, however, another variety of which my master had several vines in his garden; they are as white as our *lamparter*, and each grape is as large and as fleshy as a plum. Their size is indeed extraordinary. My mistress hung up a great number from the ceiling of my chamber for me. A single bunch was enough for a day.

On the 24th of August, Saint Bartholomew's day, the onion market is held. The onions are bound into strings with straw, and piled up like so many faggots, in piles two feet high. The whole square is covered with them, and only narrow passages are left for people to walk about. The onions are of all kinds, some very large and others white and sweet, but none of them are as strong as ours are.

On the 13th of September my master began his harvests. There is scarcely a year when it does not rain about this time, and it did not miss on this occasion. The autumn is in general more rainy than the winter.

On the 14th of September I had a very inflamed eye. Louis, one of the assistant pharmacists, when closing a sack of powder, had blown some of the dust into my eyes. But it did not have any ill consequences. I instilled *oleum gariophillorum*, which I had just learned to prepare.

When I was in the pharmacy in the evening of the 27th of September, I saw a man enter who was dressed like a German, with a small round hat, like those worn by children in those days. He came up to me and greeted me politely. It was Henry Pantaléon, the former curate of Saint Peter's, in Basel, and a professor at the *pedagogium*. I was astonished to see him here. He spoke Latin to everyone, believing that all Frenchmen understood that language. I took him to my lodging and asked what he was doing in this town. This is the story he told me. He had suffered an injustice: the living of Saint Peter's had been given to a pastor from Arüw, although this appointment belonged to him by right, as curate; further, was he not a licentiate in theology? This was true, for I had myself seen that degree conferred on him in Basel. This injustice had caused him to resign his position as curate. However, he had really little taste for the profession of preaching—he preferred the bottle, good company, and amusements. Since then he had thought of turning to medicine, and had assiduously attended the lectures of Doctor Albanus Thorinus, and read the works of Fuchsius. He had abandoned theology and theologians and gone to study for his doctorate in Valence. From that town he had come on to Montpellier, to see the country and also to visit Pézenas, where he hoped to collect some money that was owed to him.

Pantaléon's story surprised both me and my friends Myconius and Hummel, to whom I recounted it. We invited him to supper at the College. Other Germans came to keep him company. In the morning we gave him breakfast, and I remember that when he saw ripe figs being served, he asked if these were pomegranates. We gave him partridges to eat. 'Ah!' he said, 'if only my wife' (he talked of her continually) 'could eat such food!' After supper a wandering musician came by. We played him for his songs, and he lost; he was therefore obliged to sing them to us, which he did, sitting on the sill of a window. These singers know some very pretty airs, for example 'A la chambre', etc. Doctor Pantaléon marvelled and vowed that he had never heard anything so beautiful. Myconius took him by the arm. 'You astonish me,' he said, 'for you were a great fellow for songs in your younger days.' Pantaléon laughed.

He asked us to take him to Villeneuve, and to show him the sea, where he gathered quantities of shells. Our celebrated poet Lotichius was with us. Pantaléon begged him to improvise some verses on the way, and said: '*Germani socii tendunt ad littora maris.*' 'Not *maris,*' Lotichius replied, 'quia prima brevis, sed ponti.'[31] Afterwards

Pantaléon sang the *'Knight of Steuermark'* for us, from beginning to end, and was gay and happy throughout the day. In the morning he left for Pézenas, to get his money, but he got nothing. Jacob Hugguelin went with him, and caught some illness on the journey.

Doctor Pantaléon had brought a letter from my father, who bade me take care when bathing in the sea, and reminded me of the danger I had once encountered in Basel, when I had been bathing in the Birse and had nearly been dragged down into the Rhine. He said that the lute-player Theobald Schoenauer had returned from Italy and was once more lodged with him, and taught the lute to the boarders, as he had done before. He added that two companies of men had left Basel for France, under the command of Bernhard Stehelin, host of the *Golden Head* and lately made a knight, of Hütche, and of Wilhelm Hepdenring. A battle had been fought between Albert of Brandenburg and Maurice of Saxony, who had been shot and had died three days afterwards. The King of England had been poisoned.[32] My father once more urged me to work well, and to consider that there were already many doctors in Basel, without counting medical students, of whom he gave me details. Doctor Pantaléon also wished to establish himself in Basel, and so augment the already large number of practitioners there. He also had something to say of Gilbert Catalan, who did much as he wished in the house, and whose flirtations led him into a thousand follies.

On the 4th of October Pantaléon left for home, and I took advantage of the opportunity to write to my father. On the 6th Petrus Lotichius also left, with his disciples Erhardus Stibare and Conradus Demerus; they went to Avignon.

Guillaume Dalençon of Mountauban, a former priest, was unfrocked on the 16th of October. He had turned protestant and had brought some books back with him from Geneva. He had been in prison for a long time. Dressed in his priestly robes, he was brought on to a platform before the bishop. After protracted ceremonies in Latin he was divested of his chasuble and the rest, and given secular clothing. His head was then shaved, and two fingers were cut off his hand. After this he was delivered to the civil justice and once more thrown into prison.

The professors recommenced their lectures on Saint Luke's day, the 18th of October. They had ceased to teach during the summer, except for a few professors who had conducted private courses for extra fees.

On the 6th of November I sent a quantity of fruit and seeds to Basel, and I followed up this consignment with a letter to say that the Turkish fleet had arrived off Aigues Mortes, and that we had perceived it plainly at sea. The King of France had concluded an alliance with the Turks.

Johann Zonion, of Ravenspurg, came to Montpellier on the 9th of December. A schoolmaster in Little Basel, he had married a woman of seventy, who had given him money to enable him to study medicine in France. After her death he returned to practice in Ravenspurg.

He brought me a long letter from my father, and others from other persons. My father once more recommended the advantages of study and piety. I should need exceptional knowledge to succeed in Basel among so many doctors, both young and old. He told me that he had sold his printing house to Louis Lucius, but that the latter had not kept his side of the bargain, and the printing house was once more in my father's hands. In his school he had put on his famous German comedy, in which I should have played the title role of Bromius, host of the *Dead Tree*; Gilbert had taken my part. All the notabilities of the town had been present, and had done my father great honour. Herr Binningen, the Hollander, who turned out to be no other than David Georgius[33] in disguise, had offered a prize of a golden crown. Among items of political news, he told me that Albert, the Marquis of Brandenburg, was at war with the Bishop of Nuremberg. I had told him of my progress with the lute and he complimented me on it.

On the 11th of December Frederick Rihener, Hugguelin, and I went through the street, playing music. All three of us played the lute. The townspeople would willingly have chased us away, but in the end they left the way free for us.

Marius Stibare left on the 14th of December, and I gave him a letter for Lotichius. I met Stibare again, in Stuttgart, where he had become physician to the landgrave, Ludwig of Hesse; he afterwards became a professor at Heidelberg.

On the 14th of November there was an anatomy session. The subject was an old man, whose lungs were in a very bad state. Maître Guichardus presided.

On the 6th of January Guillaume Dalençon, unfrocked eleven weeks before, and since then held in prison, was condemned to death. In the afternoon a man carried him on his shoulders out of the town towards the monastery[34] to the place of execution. A pyre had already been built there. Behind the condemned man two other prisoners walked, one a cloth shearer, in his shirt, with a bale of straw fastened to his back; the other of good appearance, and well dressed. Both of them had recanted and denied the true faith. Dalençon, however, sang psalms all the way. At the pyre, he sat down on a log and himself took off his clothes as far as his shirt, and arranged them beside him tidily, as though he would be putting them on again. He exhorted the other two, who were about to apostatize, so touchingly that the sweat stood out in great drops, as big as peas, on the forehead of the man in the shirt. When the monks, formed in a curve around him and mounted on horseback, told him that it was time to make an end, he leapt joyously on to the pyre and sat down at the foot of the stake that rose in the centre of it. This stake was pierced by a hole, through which ran a cord with a running noose. The executioner put the cord round Dalençon's neck, tied his hands across his breast, and placed near him the religious books he had brought from Geneva. Then he set fire to the pyre. The martyr remained seated, calm and resigned, with his eyes raised towards heaven. When the fire reached the books the executioner pulled on the cord and strangled him; his head dropped to his breast and he made no further movement. Little by little the body was reduced to cinders. His two companions stood at the foot of the fire, where they were made to watch his sufferings, and could feel the heat of the flame.

After the execution they were both taken to the Hôtel de Ville. Near there, in front of the church of Notre-Dame, a platform had been set up, with a statue of the Virgin on it, before which they would have to recant. The crowd had to wait for them for a long time. At last only one of the two men was brought out. The cloth shearer had refused to abjure and demanded that he should be executed without mercy for having failed his beliefs. He was therefore taken

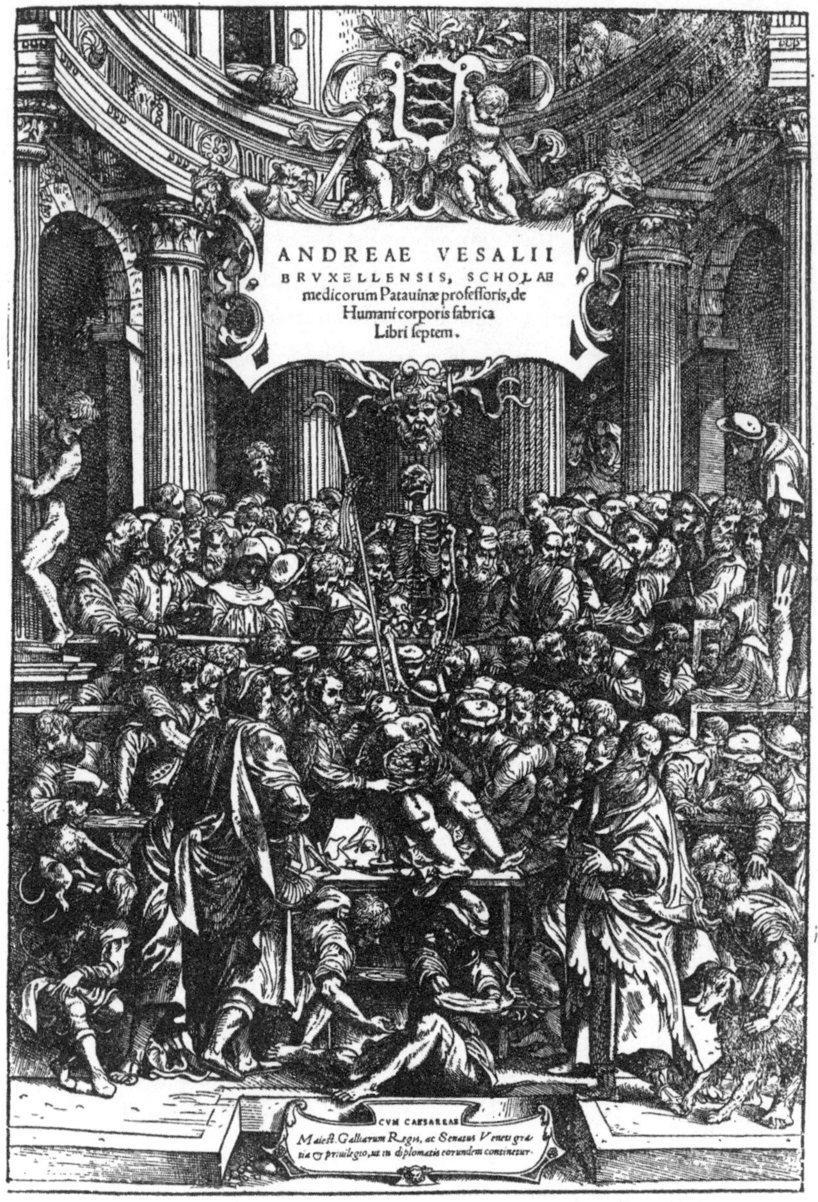

10. An anatomy theatre in the sixteenth century. A live model clings to a pillar on the left, a skeleton is in the centre, and a corpse on the table (from the title page of the works of Vesalius, printed in Basel)

back to prison. The other man, who seemed to be a man of substance, was placed on his knees before the statue of the Virgin, with a lighted candle in his hand. A clerk read out various charges, to which he had to reply. In this way he saved his life, but he was sent to the galleys and there put in chains.

On the following Tuesday, the 9th of January, it was the turn of the cloth shearer again. He was strangled and burnt as the priest had been. He showed great courage, and no less repentance for having come so near to denying his faith. It had rained on that day, and the fire would not burn. The victim, who was not completely strangled, endured great suffering. At last the monks of the neighbouring monastery brought some straw, and the executioner took it and sent for oil of terebinth from my master's pharmacy to ignite the fire. Afterwards I reproached the assistants who had given it to him, but they advised me to hold my tongue, for the same fate could befall me also, as a heretic.

During these affairs an extraordinary phenomenon occurred. On the 6th of January, immediately after the execution of the first man, it began to thunder violently. I heard it plainly and so did many others with me; but the priests derided us and said that it was the smoke from the burning of heretics that produced that effect.

On the 7th of January the wedding of Doctor Fontanonus took place. He was in a poor state of health, and quite withered and yellow, though only a young doctor. He was the son of Denys, the author of a *Pratique*. He always went about mounted on a mule, which had served his father for many years, so that, as he told me himself, it must have been more than forty years old.

According to custom the young couple were conducted to church on Sunday evening, in a procession with numerous torches and musical instruments, and afterwards were taken home in the same manner. After the meal, and while everyone was dancing, with the doors open, a Monsieur Le Beau presented himself. He was a young, good-looking student, who claimed to be of noble birth, and therefore always carried a sword, a thing that students did not customarily do. He was accompanied by one of his friends, a man called Miliet, a good dancer, as indeed Le Beau was, and who never missed a ball. Now, there was another student there, called Flaminius, a burly and arrogant Italian. He mocked at Le Beau, and tripped him, so that he nearly fell. Le Beau replied to this with a box on the ear. They would have fought on the spot if they had not been separated. Flaminius swore to have his revenge.

On Monday, after dinner, Le Beau was walking, as usual, on the paved Place Notre-Dame, when Flaminius came up like a madman, brandishing a dagger. Le Beau retreated and drew his sword, and presented the point, saying 'Go away, Flaminius!' But the other tried to knock up the sword and throw himself on Le Beau. Then Le Beau thrust his sword into Flaminius's chest, through and through, so that the steel showed a foot behind his back. Flaminius cried out 'I am killed!' and died at once. He was carried away on a ladder. Le Beau fled with his sword in his hand and hid in a house, but he was pursued. The bailly and his sergeants entered the house and searched it, while

Le Beau took refuge on the roof, and went from house to house. At last he was caught and taken to the prison of the Cour du Bayle,[35] where he suffered a long and severe imprisonment. In the end he obtained the king's pardon and was set free. He had never ceased to maintain that Flaminius had leapt upon his sword, and this contributed to his acquittal. Later he became a doctor in Tours, and he still lived there not many years ago.

On the 6th of January the Germans gathered at the College to draw the kings. The old beadle, who had lived for a long time in Greece, cooked for us. Andre, from Croatia, got the bean. Two days later we drew them again in Rondelet's house, where Jerome Betz, of Constance, lived, and Clusius, who was his secretary, and several other Germans. It was on this occasion that I made my first attempt at dancing in the French manner. I was familiar in the house, for I had taught the lute to Rondelet's daughter Catherine, who long after this married Doctor Salomon.

Doctor Jacob Hugguelin was spending more than his means and needed money. He sent a messenger to Basel to bring some. For this mission he chose a peasant called Antoine, whom Catalan employed frequently in his gardens. He carried letters for me to my father and to other people, and I sent home some theriaque[36] *correctam a Rondeletio*, and some of the delicious powder of violets. I asked my father to send me some strings for my lute.

On the 26th of January we were visited by two guards of the King of Navarre. One was called Jacob Heilmann, and the other Fritz, from Zurich. We made them welcome. Fritz related, among other stories, a combat between a bull and a lion, during which the bull had gored him just under the navel, and his water had gushed out of the hole; nevertheless, he had recovered, with the help of God.

On Shrove Tuesday the doctors went about the town in masks, and attacked the townspeople with a hail of oranges, as I described last year.

On the 27th Carolus Clusius left Montpellier. He was Rondelet's secretary, and was lodging with him when I arrived. In after years he made himself famous in botanical science, on account of his writings on that subject, and never practised medicine. He wrote to me often to recall our days in Montpellier.

On the 2nd of February there was another anatomy session, the subject being a man.

On the 10th a criminal was executed. He was beheaded on a scaffold, and his four limbs were cut off, as the usage is in this country.

Doctor Honoratus Castellanus began to lecture again, after a long cessation. He was very eloquent, and reminded me of T. Zwingerus.[37]

Antoine had been gone four weeks, and I began to feel impatient for his return. On the 26th of February, after dinner, I went with a friend on the road to Castelnau, beside the olive trees. Suddenly I saw a man coming in our direction: it was Antoine. He brought me good news from home, where, he said, he had been given some excellent red wine. He had brought me a thick bundle of letters, and another for Hugguelin, who had employed him. I returned home to read mine, but as supper was ready, I could not do it until we had left the table. My master read his, nevertheless. His sons said that they worked incessantly. As for me, I was so happy that I nearly ate two

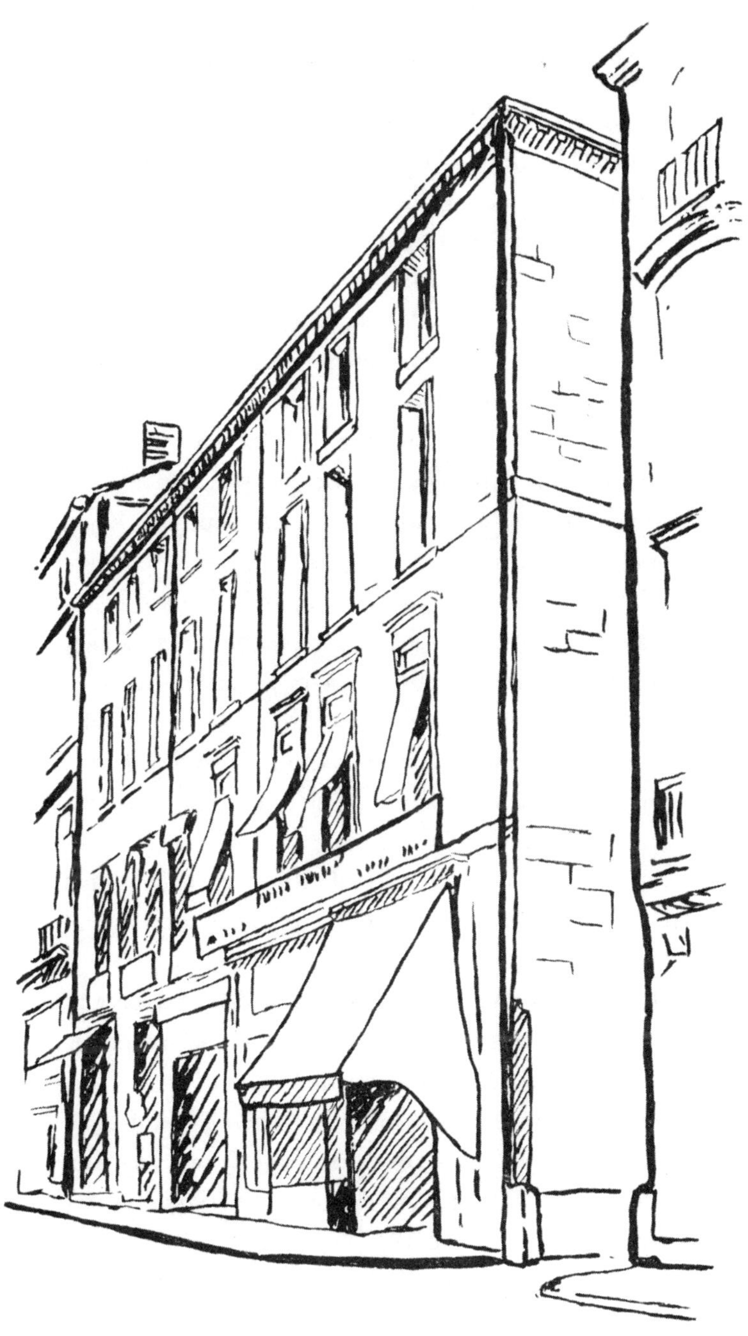

11. Rondelet's house today (drawing by Seán Jennett)

needles that had fallen into what was served to me. I was frightened by this accident, and said to myself that there is never any pleasure without pain.

After supper I read my father's letter. It was two folded sheets, filled with small, fine writing. He enjoined me to fear God, and to be honest, pious, and studious, and counselled me to apply myself especially to surgery—the number of doctors in Basel was great, and I should never be able to make my mark there if I did not show more than the usual ability. I must remember that I was the son of a poor schoolmaster, while the others came of rich and powerful families.

Theobald, the lute player, had also written to me to send me lute strings and various pieces of music. Gilbert also wrote, and told me that Doctor Pantaléon had been nicknamed Doctor Watering Can since he had told a woman complaining of insomnia to pour water over her head during the night, from a watering can. A farce had been written about it.

Antoine brought to Doctor Hugguelin the news that his mother had no money and therefore could not send him any. However, he was determined to return home, and after eight days he sent Antoine a second time to Basel, on the 5th of March. I gave him a letter for my father, whom I told how fortunate I thought I was, to be situated in my master's pharmacy, where I could learn how to prepare all kinds of remedies; for it was very well stocked. I added a prescription of Doctor Saporta's, for strengthening the memory.

On the 23rd of March a commissioner came from Toulouse, and in company with the bailly searched the town for Lutherans. At that time all reformed Christians were called by this name, and the names of Calvinist and Huguenot were unknown. It was cried throughout the town, to the sound of a trumpet, that all who knew of any must denounce them, or be themselves severely punished.

The following day the sister of the Bishop of Montpellier and her husband were burned in effigy, in the form of two clothed dummies, in the square. The woman's apron took fire and flew up high into the air, and this caused a burst of laughter from the crowd.[38]

Paul Stibare returned to Montpellier on the 27th.

On the 31st our former beadle's son was executed. He was a fine fellow, and his wife had the appearance of a lady. He used to travel about Provence, and often brought gems or coral back from his journeys. These things aroused suspicion, and it was discovered that he had been following the profession of highwayman. After this he could no longer let himself be seen in Montpellier. The thieftakers were set upon him, and they surprised him in a village, in a house, where he defended himself furiously. He was wounded several times in the head before he was captured. He was brought back wounded to Montpellier, and a few days later he was beheaded on the scaffold. After his death his limbs were cut off, as the custom is.

In the morning Antoine returned from Basel, having made the journey there and back in twenty-six days. He brought Hugguelin ninety crowns, his mother's entire fortune. Hugguelin bought a fine horse, and at once began to prepare to leave.

My father wrote that he was glad to learn from a letter sent to him by Doctor Saporta that I was making good progress in my studies. He told me that Doctor Huber had frequently declared that I should one day be a famous physician. He added that Thomas Schoepfius had been appointed physician to the town of Colmar.

Israel Nübelspach arrived from the Duchy of Baden on the 1st of April; he was a little man and was constantly drunk, when he became as red as a lobster. Johannes Desyderius, a distinguished scholar, also came.

On the 2nd two men from Constance, whom I had found in Montpellier on my arrival, returned home. They were Andreas de Croatie, who afterwards became a physician at Ravenspurg, and Paulus Stibare, of Würzburg. Peter Heel, of Kaufbeuren, went with them; he was a jolly fellow, but he was later murdered.

On the 10th, Jacob Hugguelin, Henricius and Martinas Stibare, and their tutor Georgius Fischerus, all left Montpellier. I gave them a letter for my father, in which I mentioned that I had been ill for some time with catarrh. I recommended Fischerus and the Stibare brothers to him.

On the morrow I rode to my master's farm at Vendargues, together with a group of his relatives, among whom were some young girls.

On the 16th of April I was asked by Monsieur Guichard de Sandre, who was lodged in a house opposite to me, to come and give a serenade to a lady. We went there at midnight. We began with rolls on a side drum, to awaken the inhabitants of the street; after that came the trumpets, and these were followed by hautboys. These in turn were succeeded by fifes, and then viols, and finally a trio of lutes. The serenade lasted a full hour and a half. Afterwards we went to an inn, where we were treated with magnificence and drank muscat and hippocras throughout the remainder of the night.

It was on this same day that two soldiers arrived from Piedmont. They were Jacob Schieli, a butcher from Basel, and Henri Seiler. They were both destitute and dressed in rags, and Schieli's legs were swollen and frost-bitten. We took them to the College and lighted a fire there to warm them. We gave the Basel man an old shawl, or *flassada*, of Catalan weave, such as most of the students wear, and a pair of old shoes, and some other clothes. We also gave them money, as well as a good supper. Schieli wept for joy, 'I shall go happily on my way,' he said, 'since I am now so well fed.'

On the 18th of April two very different men from Basel came to Montpellier. They were soldiers of the King of Navarre, and of splendid appearance, in their fine slashed clothes and with their arms and halberds. They were Johann Brombach, a barber, and Johann Pfriendt, a butcher, and they were on their way home. After we had taken them round the town, we invited them to supper with us. In Basel they had shown themselves enemies of the students there, and had often fought with them at night; but they were so won over by our good reception of them that they promised henceforward to take the students' part, instead of fighting against them. We went with them as far as Castelnau. There we drank a stirrup cup, and to mark the engagement into which they had entered, they were baptized with a glass of wine, which was poured over their heads.

On the 21st of April Frederick Rihener, my bedfellow, left Montpellier for Salers, in Limousin, where his brother had a house. We accompanied him on the way, as far as a neighbouring village, where we stayed to drink together until late in the evening. At last he mounted his horse and went off, and we returned to the town. Unfortunately he lost his way, and after wandering about all night found himself in the morning back in the village where we had taken leave of him. He sent us word of his misadventure, and some of us went at once to join him, and sat drinking with him until he left once more.

In May we went to the sea to bathe. When I came out of the water I buried myself in the warm sand, and three days afterwards I had catarrh. I purged myself for it.

On the 22nd of May Stephen Contzenus, of Bern, returned from Strasbourg to Montpellier and brought me a letter from my father. In it my father told me that several Basel students had married: Wildicius, later pastor at Liestal, had married Dorothy, a dressmaker; Materne Vach had married the aged Wildicia, Wildicius's mother; Pedionaeus, his headmaster, had married Pellonius's sister; and Bartholomew Schindler had married an old woman. My father also said that on the 28th of April three companies of men had left Basel for France under the command of Bernhard Stehelin and Huschen. He returned once more to the number of doctors in Basel. '*Nisi excellueris, esuriendum tibi erit*', he said, that is to say, if I did not prove an exceptional man, then I should die of hunger. Batt Haler, my school friend, had behaved badly and had been banished from the town. He was an only son, and as such had been too much indulged. He was a merry fellow, and loved nothing but to be entertained. When he was a student he had no care in his head but to play the lute and to run after every pretty girl, and to join in every jest and masquerade. He ended by promising marriage to a young dressmaker called Muntzinger, from Little Basel. He married her, too, and had two children by her, Beatus and Jacob, who became good men when they grew up, because they scarcely knew their father and were brought up in their grandfather's house. Despite his marriage Batt continued with his former way of life, and began to court Gorius Wentz's daughter in law, who lived on the wheat market, at the sign of the 'Salmon'. She was called little Annette of the 'Salmon'.[39] They would dance sometimes in the house, late, on Catalonian carpets, so that the neighbours should not be disturbed in the night. Eventually the girl became pregnant, and was put in prison with her mother, who was considered to be an accomplice in the matter. The child was baptized. The mother was banished, and went to Schliengen, where she married no less than three times, and I believe that she lives there still in this year 1612. The seducer fled to Lorraine. There he fell in love with a nun at Rimelsberg, of the house of Tinterville, if I am not mistaken, and ran away with her. They were pursued, and the girl was caught. He was not caught until long afterwards. Then, while he was being carried chained in a cart, and being taken across a river, the vehicle overturned and the prisoner was drowned. No one knows whether it really was an accident.

On the 25th of June Jerome Popius left. He was a Strasbourger, and had been in Montpellier when I arrived. He went to establish himself as a physician in Strasbourg, where he died. A number of us accompanied him as far as Lunel, and in the morning we went on as

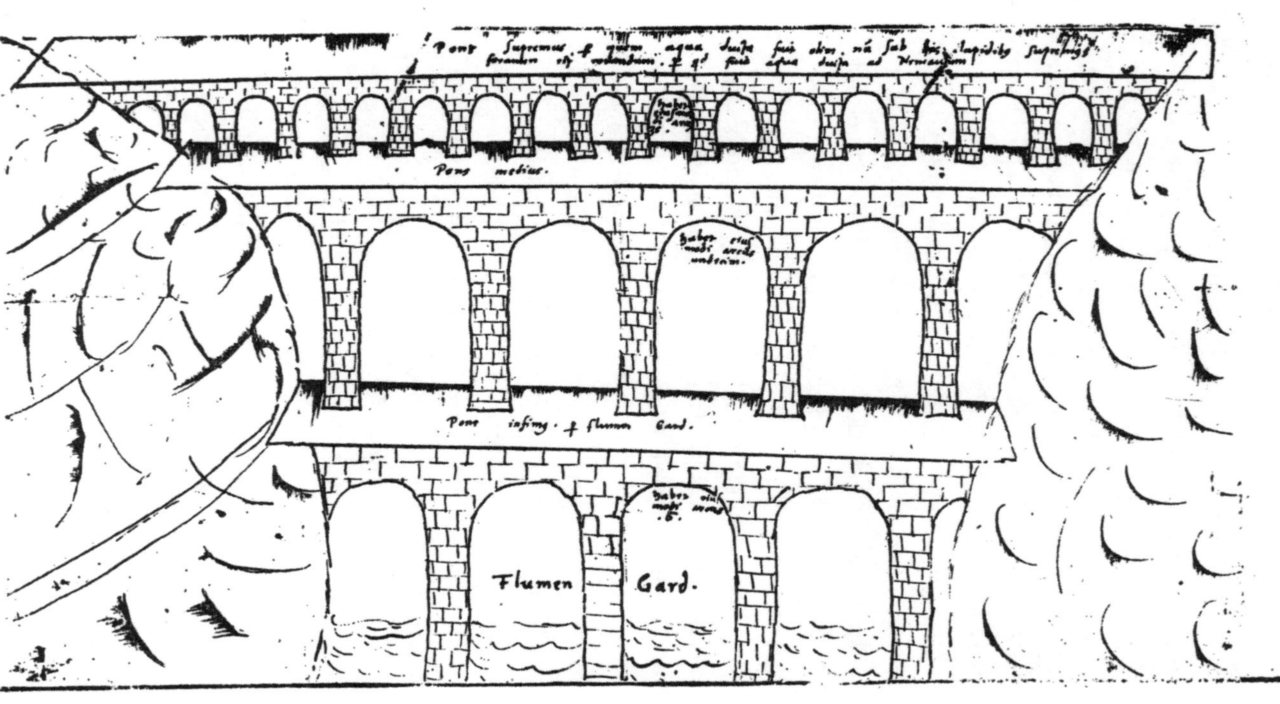

12. Felix Platter's drawing of the Pont du Gard (taken from the journal)

far as Nîmes to see the antiquities and the amphitheatre, which is immense. I saw again the sculptured group of Romulus and Remus being suckled by a she-wolf, and the statue of a man with three faces. We left Nîmes to sleep in Sernhac, so that in the morning we might go and see the famous Pont du Gard; it is a wonderful structure, of three stages, of which the first has six arches, the second eleven, and the third thirty-six. It is built of huge dressed stones, and is of prodigious height, joining two mountains. At the very top there is a covered channel, through which water flows. Here is the drawing that I made of it at that time.

In the evening I went to Avignon, and in the morning I paced the length of the stone bridge that crosses the Rhône: it measures 1,300 paces.[40] In the middle there is a chapel. The bridge is paved with small white flagstones, so slippery that it is dangerous to cross on horseback—you must lead your horse by the bridle. A proverb says that no one crosses without meeting two monks, two donkeys, and two whores. Because they pay large dues, the latter are protected by the authorities in this town. They live in two long streets, in which they occupy all the houses. They may be seen before their doors, very richly dressed, and they invite the passer-by to enter, and even go so far as to stop him. They say that their leader, who is derisively called the 'abbess', is obliged to give herself for nothing to any student who asks.

There is a university in the town where the degree of doctor is conferred.

The palace was formerly the residence of the Popes. At the top of this château we were shown an iron cage in which a protestant had been imprisoned and exposed to all weathers until he died.

In the evening I returned to Nîmes, and on the following day came once more to Montpellier, after an absence of five days. On the 8th of July I had a singular dream. I dreamed that I consulted a barber in Basel for a pain in the hand. The barber's daughter applied a remedy that assuaged my suffering at once. She was no other than my future wife. I divined from this that my wedding could not be far away.

On the 2nd of August I wrote to my father, and sent my letter by a merchant who was going to the fair at Lyon. I told him that Doctor Saporta had talked with me, and would himself tell him the result. I was practising distilling. I was writing down many prescriptions that I got from the doctors, and I had copied out others from Falcon's writings, which my master kept shut up in a room of the house he had inherited from that physician. I had got into this room by way of a ladder, and not without danger. I also told him about my journey to the Pont du Gard.

As in the previous year I went on the 10th of August with Hummel and Myconius to see my master's vine. We ate a great quantity of grapes, for they were very abundant, in bunches of extraordinary size.

On the 19th of August we received a visit from two gentlemen, who stayed for some time. They were J. Morenholdt and J. Burck. Benedictus Burgauwer, of Lindau, arrived about this time; he was afterwards a physician in Schaff house.

On the 26th, as a number of Germans were accompanying one of their number home with torches, after supper, they were arrested by the captain of the watch and his sergeants, who took their swords and daggers from several of them. It caused a great tumult in front of my master's pharmacy, where I was just then. We ran out to see what was going on. Stephen Contzenus obstinately refused to give up his dagger to the captain. Monsieur Catalan intervened and asked him to surrender the dagger to him. Contzenus allowed himself to be persuaded, and the clamour died down. In the morning, however, he protested to the bailly and complained about this infringement of the privileges that had been accorded to Germans. The captain was admonished, and we were promised that nothing of the kind should happen again.

On the 4th of September 1554 I received a letter from my father, who had been made anxious by my long silence. Lotichius[41] and Fischerus had been to see him, and had told him that I was doing well. Lotichius sent me his good wishes as a fellow of the pen. He had been in the habit of calling me by this name in Montpellier, and for this reason. Not long after I came there I was in the College, composing Latin verses. Lotichius came to sit by me. He was a distinguished poet, but I knew nothing of that. He read my verses and told me that I really must teach him how to do it. I agreed, and demonstrated some of the rules. When the other Germans got to know about this, they made fun of me, and told me that Lotichius had lately been acclaimed as a master of Latin versification, and had even published a book of verses at Lyon. I went at once in search of him and reproached him. 'You have made a fool of me,' I said. 'How, a fool?' he asked. 'Yes, a fool, chatterbox,' I said. 'Chatterbox, no,' he answered, 'but a fellow scribbler, that I agree,' and thereafter he never called me otherwise.

On the 18th of September Eléonore, Catalan's wife, gave birth to a daughter, who was called Anna. This was the second child she had had while I was in the house.

On the 21st three Germans left Montpellier. They were Andreas Bury, Antonius Zitwitz, and Gregorius Zimmermann.

On the 28th the Provost came to Montpellier, and there were several executions. On the first day he appeared on horseback, preceded by several horsemen and followed by the town trumpeter sounding his trumpet. Behind him walked a criminal, with some monks. He was a handsome young man and had been an accomplice in a murder. He was brought to a scaffold that had been erected in front of the Hôtel de Ville. There a Saint Andrew's cross had been made with two hollowed-out balks of timber; in this his limbs were to be broken. The condemned man stood and recounted in rhyme the crime he had committed, and at the end he added: 'Pray to Holy Mary that she may intercede with her Son to take me into Paradise.' The executioner then undressed him and tied him by the limbs to the cross, as those are tied, with us, who are to be broken on the wheel. Then he took a heavy bar of iron, called a massa, sharpened a little on one side, and broke the man's limbs with it. This punishment resembles our punishment of the wheel, and is called here *massarrer.* The last blow was struck on the chest, and this killed the victim.

On the next day a false coiner was hanged in the same place. The gibbet was not very high and had only one arm.

Afterwards a masked dummy was brought on a hurdle, and was laid on the cross and its limbs broken, as I have described. This dummy represented a Greek who had studied at Montpellier and had been accounted one of the keenest blades of the town. He had married Gillette d'Andrieu, a girl of doubtful reputation, who had neither beauty nor fortune. She had a very long nose, and her lover could scarcely manage to kiss her on the lips, especially since he too had a nose of respectable size. The Greek was insulted by a canon, Pierre Saint-Ravy, who taunted him, at the moment when he was about to relieve himself, of having had intercourse with his wife. The husband at once stabbed the canon and fled; he could therefore be executed only in effigy. His wife continued to live in Montpellier, and was often in Rondelet's house—she was a relative of his. She often came there to dance, and one day I danced with her, all booted and spurred, on my return from Vendargues. As I turned. my spurs entangled themselves in her dress, and I fell full length on the floor. Some tablets I had in a breast pocket were broken into pieces, and I was so stunned that I had to be helped up.

On the 4th of November I received a letter from my father. He spoke at length of a desire he had formed to print Falcon's 'Practica', on whatever condition his widow might impose. He said that Thomas Guerin, on his way back from the fair at Frankfurt, had been robbed by brigands led by the innkeeper of the *Eagle* at Laufenberg. Guerin denounced him later in Basel, and he fled on foot. His horse was taken and was sold by auction. A merchant from Geneva lost his wife in the robbery, which took place at Besen, near Brisach.

On Sunday the 11th of November we celebrated the engagement of my master's elder daughter Isabelle to the son of a merchant of Béziers, who was also a Maran. The ceremony took place in the great salon of the house in which I lived. The dancing went on in a long room where we sat at a table so narrow that one's knees touched those of the person opposite. There were several Maran maidens, and among them was Jeanne de Sos, daughter of the physician Pierre de Sos. She was a young girl and very amiable, and she was so charming to me, both in the dance and in conversation, that I almost lost my head. Afterwards she married Doctor Saporta, after he had lost his first wife. I remember that one day she ate so many chestnuts that she had to be given an enema. Her fiancé went home, but left with his future wife one of his sisters, a little rounded woman full of good nature and kindness.

I lived quite alone in Catalan's house after Frederic left, but after supper, which we always ate in the pharmacy, Hummel would come with me, so that I should not have to sleep alone. He would bring almonds to persuade me to play the lute to him. Sometimes other Germans would come, especially Myconius, for he liked to drink a cup of wine before going to bed. I had the key of the cellar, about which my master did not concern himself, since the wine in this country keeps only a year. One day one of us got into a locked cellar by sliding under the door. He found hippocras there, and we passed a jug to him to be filled, but it would not come back upright under the door, and we had to empty it into goblets. When this was done, we pulled him back under the door. Altogether, we committed many youthful follies.

Catalan had a quantity of dried grapes hung up in a room. We found a way of hooking them out with a long pole through a hole in the eaves. We took care to throw the stalks back into the room, and Catalan was firmly convinced that his grapes had been eaten by rats. It was wicked of us, it must be admitted.

On the 14th I sent a box to Lyon, to be consigned to Basel. It contained Falcon's 'Opus practicam',[42] which was to be printed in Basel on condition that a hundred crowns were to be paid to the widow. I also enclosed two langoustes without claws, and an enormous crab, as big as a plate, and quite dried up. There was also a leaf of the Indian fig for my father to plant; it came from the one that I grew in a vase on the roof, and which had flourished and put out several leaves. One of these plants in my master's garden had become a real tree, with several branches, and produced fruit; nevertheless it had grown from a single leaf from Italy. Further, I included a quantity of shells, as well as ninety-five large pomegranates, some sweet and some acid, which I had bought in the market, all except a few given by Antoine; also sixty-three beautiful oranges, a basket of dried grapes, and some figs, of which my father gave some away and kept the rest. Finally there was a large pot of compounded mithridate and a small skeleton, and a letter.

Near All Souls' Day Rondelet presided at an autopsy at which a monkey was dissected. The liver and spleen were covered with pustules filled with water, which burst at the slightest touch. Those on the liver were reddish in colour, except for those in the region of the bile vessel, which tended to be yellow. I thought that the animal had died of dropsy. Some days afterwards there was another session, at which the subject was a handsome courtesan who had died in childbirth. Her womb was still swollen, since the delivery had only recently occurred.

On the 16th of November a German sent Antoine to Strasbourg in search of money. I gave him a letter for my father, whom I told that the Turks had landed with twenty-five galleys at Aigues Mortes, and with eighteen others at Frontignan, the country of the muscat. It was thought that they would make their winter quarters there, and this caused some disquiet, for they had a great deal of artillery and were very well equipped.

I had always desired to know everything concerning medicine, even those parts commonly neglected. I was mindful, too, of the multitude of physicians in Basel, among whom I could make my way only by superior knowledge. I could not expect to be assisted by my father, who was overwhelmed with debt, had only a small income, and was reduced to living on what revenue came from the boarders in his school. I could not have imagined then that he would remarry in his old age and have a large number of children. The desire to learn made me follow with attention not only the lectures and ordinary studies, but also the preparation of remedies in the pharmacy, a matter I found very useful later. Further, I collected plants, and arranged them properly on paper. But my principal study was anatomy. Not only did I never miss the dissections of men and animals that took place in the College, but I also took part in every secret autopsy of corpses, and I came to put my own hand to the scalpel, despite the repulsion I had felt at first. I joined with French students and exposed myself to danger to procure subjects. A bachelor of medicine named Gallotus, who had married a woman from Montpellier and was passing rich, would lend us his house. He invited me, with some others, to join him in nocturnal expeditions outside the town, to dig up bodies freshly buried in the cloister cemetery, and we carried them to his house for dissection. We had spies to tell us of burials and to lead us by night to the graves.

Our first excursion of this kind took place on the 11th of November 1554. As night fell Gallotus led us out of the town to the monastery of the Augustins, where we met a monk, called Brother Bernhard, a determined fellow, who had disguised himself in order to help us. When we came to the monastery[43] we stayed to drink, quietly, until midnight. Then, in complete silence, and with swords in hand, we made our way to the cemetery of the monastery of Saint-Denis.[44] There we dug up a corpse with our hands, the earth being still loose, because the burial had taken place only that day. As soon as we had uncovered it we pulled it out with ropes, wrapped it in a *flassada*, and carried it on two poles as far as the gates of the town. It must then have been about three o'clock in the morning. We put the corpse to one side and knocked on the postern that is opened for coming and going at night, and the old porter came in his shirt to open it for us. We asked him to bring us something to drink, under the pretext that we were dying of thirst, and while he went in search of wine three of us brought the cadaver in and carried it directly to Gallotus's house, which was not far away. The porter was not suspicious, and we rejoined our companions. On opening the winding sheet in which the body was sewn, we found a woman with a congenital deformity of the legs, the two feet turned inwards. We did an autopsy and found, among other curiosities, various veins *vasorum spermaticorum*, which were not deformed, but followed the curve of the legs towards the buttocks. She had a lead ring, and as I detest these it added to my disgust.

Encouraged by the success of this expedition, we tried again five days later. We had been informed that a student and a child had been buried in the same cemetery of Saint-Denis. When night came we left the town to go to the monastery of the Augustins. It was the 16th of December. In Brother Bernhard's cell we ate a chicken cooked with cabbage. We got the cabbage ourselves, from the garden, and seasoned it with wine supplied by the monk. Leaving the table, we went out with our weapons drawn, for the monks of Saint-Denis had discovered that we had exhumed the woman, and they had threatened us direly should we return. Myconius carried his naked sword, and the Frenchmen their rapiers. The two corpses were disinterred, wrapped in our cloaks, and carried on poles as before as far as the gates of the town. We did not dare to rouse the porter this time, so one of us crawled inside through a hole that we discovered under the gate—for they were very negligently maintained. We passed the cadavers through the same opening, and they were pulled through from the inside. We followed in turn, pulling ourselves through on our backs; I remember that I scratched my nose as I went through.

The two subjects were carried to Gallotus's house and their coverings were removed. One was a student whom we had known. The autopsy revealed serious lesions. The lungs were decomposed and stank horribly, despite the

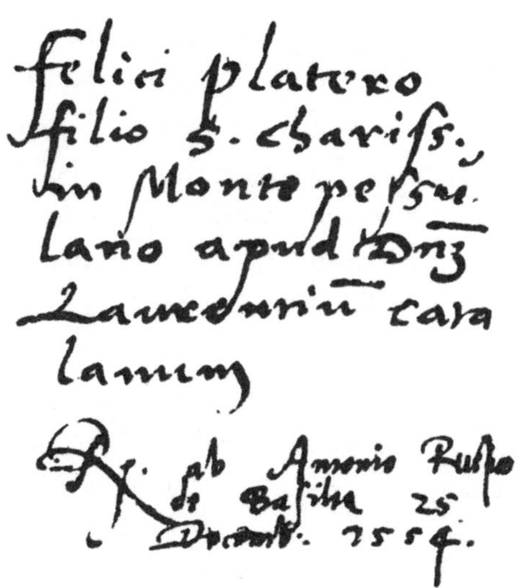

Felici platero
filio s. chariss.
in Monte pessu-
lano apud Dnz
Laurentiu cata-
lanum

R. ab Amonio Ruffo
de Basilea 25
Decemb. 1554.

13. The address on the letter, with Felix's methodical annotation of the date received and the name of the bearer (from the original in the library of the University of Basel)

vinegar that we sprinkled on them; we found some small stones in them. The child was a little boy, and we made a skeleton of him.

When I returned to my lodging early in the morning, the shop boy who slept with me did not hear me ring, and he did not wake even when I threw stones against the shutters. I was obliged to go for some sleep to the house of one of the Frenchmen who had been with us. After this the monks of Saint-Denis guarded their graveyard, and if a student came near he was received with bolts from a crossbow.

A further letter came from my father on the 5th of December, yet again exhorting me to work hard. Coelius Secundus Curio wrote to me at the same time and sent me his son's compliments. Gilbert Catalan also wrote, sending me a letter full of his love for the young girl I spoke of before; with some fine Latin verses in which he expressed his passion, and also his fears concerning me, for he imagined that I might let the cat out of the bag.

Antoine returned from Strasbourg on Christmas Day, and brought me another letter from my father, dated the 10th of December. He had come from Basel to Montpellier in fifteen days. He also brought me letters from Sebastian Castalion, Doctor Hugguelin, and others.

After New Year's Day the balls and the masquerades began again. I took part in them now, for I had learned the French dances and become a good musician. We disguised ourselves so that we could go with other revellers to the various houses in which there was dancing.

About this time we rode out again to my master's farm at Vendargues.

On the 7th of January 1555 my comrade Balthazar Hummel left to go home to Basel. I gave him various letters, including one for my father, whom I told that the Count de la Chambre, of Savoy, who had been pronounced leprous and incurable in Basel, where he had gone for treatment to the *Wild Man*, had lately been cured in Montpellier. I had noted what remedies had been used, and every day I saw cures quite as wonderful. I described how we had exhumed bodies for practice in anatomy, and I asked him to send me twenty-five crowns per year for my personal expenses. I said that he should not be too deeply concerned about the payment of his debts, for I was determined, with God's help, no longer to be a burden on him when I returned to Basel. He must not worry about my conduct, nor should he fear that I might marry a Frenchwoman, as Doctor

Henry Rihener had done, because my thoughts were fixed in Basel. I told him that before I came to Montpellier an Austrian named Zisel had married one of Rondelet's sisters called Catherine; after having led her to the altar, he left with her for Austria, but abandoned her at Lyon, telling the merchant who was his master that she was merely his mistress. The poor woman returned to Montpellier, and lived there as a widow with her brother, a pharmacist, all the time that I was in the town. The husband was killed by the Turks in Hungary.

On the 17th of January there was another anatomy session in the College. The subject was a young workman.

On the 31st we made another expedition to the cemetery outside the town. We dug up an old woman and a child and took the bodies to the Augustin monastery, to Brother Bernhard's cell, where we dissected them, for it was no longer possible to take corpses into the town. The other Germans fell out with me because I did not tell them that we were going on these expeditions, a thing I could not do because the French had made me promise, on oath, not to talk of them to anyone. On the 2nd of February I struck a bargain with my lame shoemaker, whom we called Vulcan: every Sunday he would bring me a new pair of shoes, for which I would pay him three francs yearly, which amounts to ten of our *batzen*, and he would take back the old shoes. We wore only shoes with thin soles—I have never had any with double soles. When it rained, or in winter, we wore mules over these *escarpins*.

I often saw, in front of the shoemaker's shop, a man in a long cloak, who had had his nose cut off and who dragged himself along painfully on two crutches. He had been a handsome fellow once, a writer in Nîmes, and had been the lover of the wife of a doctor of law named Bigottas. The husband, with several masked students, surprised the young man in bed with the wife. They strangled him with a cord, and after cutting off his genitals and his nose, threw him thus mutilated into the street. The victim recovered from his wounds, however, and came to Montpellier to drag out the remainder of his wretched life.[45]

On the 23rd a malefactor was executed on a scaffold in front of the chamber of the Consulat. His head was cut off, and then his four limbs, and these were hung, as usual, on olive-trees outside the town.

On this same day Lampertus, Lafferus, Gochius, and his friend Petrus left Montpellier.

On the 28th Antoine, the gardener, who had already made three journeys to Germany, was once more sent to Strasbourg. I gave him a letter for my father, whom I told that the redness that had afflicted my eyes and nose since my childhood had disappeared, despite the fact that the heat in the Midi was much greater than in Basel. I also wrote to Doctor Hugguelin to give him some information that he had asked for in his last letter. I told him that the girls whom Lotichius had called 'Sidera' were now married, including the one on whom he had doted so much because she resembled a girl he had loved at Virtemberg, and whom he called *tunicatam*[46] in his verses. She had married a doctor of law from Auvergne, and Mademoiselle Pouillane someone from Avignon.

On the 3rd of March Guillaume Heroard received the degree of doctor of medicine. He was the brother of the surgeon Michel who had accompanied me from Geneva to Montpellier. He had been on a long voyage into Sicily. Doctor Saporta presided at the ceremony, which was held in the church of Saint-Firmin, and which was conducted with great pomp, to the sound of the organ. The recipient made his speech of thanks in five or six languages, including German, although it was evident that he scarcely knew how to speak that tongue. He was led solemnly around the town to the sound of fifes, with a plume of silk on his biretta. Stalks of fennel ornamented with little figures of sugar were carried in the procession. When we returned there was a grand repast, with an abundant supply of sugared almonds—more than a quintal[47] of them. The hippocras was delicious. The repast was followed by dancing.

Antoine came back from Strasbourg on the 8th of April, bringing me a letter from my father with the news of the death of the old soap merchant[48] from Munich and his wife. He told me that the people of Solothurn had tried to seize part of the bishopric, after the death of their bishop, but that they had not been successful. He begged me not to risk myself any further in the exhumation of bodies, but none the less not to cease to gather all the medical knowledge that I could, and reminded me again that there were seventeen medical men in Basel, some already doctors and others about to become so. It would be a great advantage to be able to prepare remedies myself, as his master Doctor Epiphanius had done and got great benefit by it. As a good dancer, and also a good musician, I must be on my guard against the seductions of French women, the more so because, when I returned, there would be someone waiting for me with whom I should not be disappointed. He confided to me, in fact, that he had long ago suggested to Franz Jeckelmann that a marriage might be arranged between his daughter and me, and that he had made no objection, adding only that the matter must be left in God's hands until I returned. My father praised the girl as accomplished, honest, and devout. He had noticed long ago that I had an inclination towards her, and this had been confirmed by what Balthazar Hummel had told him, and it was for this reason that he had broached the matter with me sooner than he would otherwise have done. I should therefore turn all my thoughts in that direction, and hasten the completion of my studies, that I might the sooner return to Basel. Doctor Saporta had had a great deal of good to say about me, and had added that he was ready to confer on me a baccalaureate in medicine. My father acknowledged the receipt of the box that I had sent him, including the works of Falcon.[49] Unfortunately no one in Basel would print the book, not even for two hundred crowns, because it was half in Latin and half in French. It had therefore been decided to send it back to Lyon. He announced that Gilbert Catalan would return to Montpellier in the winter, and that I must beware of him because he was a thorough good-for-nothing, full of conceit on account of his title as a bachelor, without common sense, spendthrift, proud—such was his portrait.

By the same messenger my father sent me two beautiful skins, tinted green, of which I had an excellent suit made, embroidered with green silk. I paraded in it at the ball, and aroused the admiration of every man, for leather breeches were then quite unknown in that country. The tailor had made them a little tight, claiming that he had not had enough leather, but I found afterwards that he had robbed me of a good-sized piece and had made a bag out of it for his wife.

Hummel wrote to give me all kinds of news. Doctor Isaac Keller had married a noblewoman, and the wedding had been very grand. Doctor Hugguelin had become physician to the Marquis de Durlach; and Nicolas Meier, who, so it was said, had been my rival for the hand of my fiancée, had just died, which relieved me of some care.

I also received a letter from Theobald, the lute-player, with some strings for my lute. He had returned from Auvergne, where he had not stayed long. Attracted by the fine promises of a gentleman there, he had gone to join his household, only to find, when he arrived at the château, that the man had just been murdered by his own servants. Theobald had to return to Basel, and was giving lessons on the lute to several of my father's boarders.

In addition I received two letters from Strasbourg—one from my cousin Laurentius, and the other from Johann Odratzheim, who had been my companion in the pharmacy.

On the 16th of April Conrad Forerus, of Winterthür, and Johannes Zonion, who had married an old woman in Basel, left us. The first became a pastor in Winterthür, and performed the functions of that office at the same time as those of medicine. The second soon lost his aged wife and returned to his own district of Ravenspurg.

On the 22nd Michael Hoffman of Hall and Israel Nebelspach of Baden also left Montpellier.

On the 23rd of April I wrote to my father, principally concerning the question of my marriage. My one desire, I told him, was to receive the hand of the girl he had chosen for me, as soon as I had obtained my doctorate, that is to say, in two years' time. But the consent of her father would not be enough for me; I also desired that of the girl herself, for I wanted to marry only a woman who loved me. I begged him, therefore, to discover what were her sentiments, and also to find out what was her age, since several people had said that she was older than I was, and likely to be married before I returned.

I replied also to Theobald Schoenauer to thank him for the lute strings, and I sent him in return some pieces of music, so that he might judge the progress that I had made on the lute.

Ulricus Giger, or Chelius, the son of Doctor Giger, arrived on the 9th of May. He came from Strasbourg, and afterwards became a physician in that town. My father had given him a letter for me, but he had been wrecked while descending the Rhône, between Lyon and Avignon, and all his baggage, including letters, had been lost. He was lucky to have escaped with his life, for six of his companions and five horses had been drowned. I persuaded my master to take him as a boarder, for I lived alone in the Falcon house at that time, and I should be glad to have a companion. On the same day Theodore Birkmannus arrived from Cologne; he was a young but knowledgeable, and a clever musician. It was with him that I later travelled through France.

On the 17th of May Doctor Saporta lost his wife. His students were present when she was buried.

On the 20th of May a *disputatio quodlibetaria* began. This is what a candidate for a licentiate had to undergo. It lasted several days, and I myself posed some problems to the candidate, though I was the only one among the

Germans to do so. On the 29th of May I purged myself with *pillulas coccias*, which sent me to stool sixteen times and left me very weak. My master was sent for and was very alarmed. Nonetheless, I felt better by dinner, though I could not take my place at the table, and my meal was sent up to me in my bedchamber. While I was eating I heard singing in the street. It proved to be a Companion of Saint James,[50] and I had him brought up to me and asked him his name and his country. He was called Franz Müller, and came from Hesingen, near Basel. After giving him food and drink, I presented him with three *batzen* in

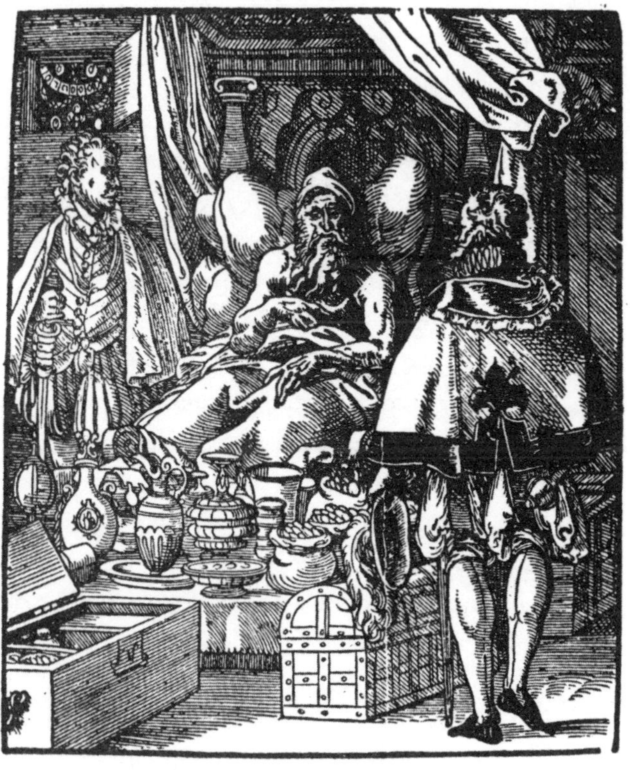

14. A doctor visiting his patient (woodcut by Jost Amman)

change, together with a box of theriaque, which he could sell on the way. I also confided a letter to his care, and he delivered it safely to my father.

Early on the morning of the 4th of June we went botanizing on the seashore, and the following evening I took part in a serenade, in which there were three of us, all lute players.

On the 19th Casparus Wolfius arrived from Zurich. He later became a physician in that town.

On the 4th of June Honoré Castellan[51] gave a grand banquet, and he asked me to play the lute behind the tapestry, which I did. He liked me very well, often took me with him on his medical visits, and frequently invited me to dinner at his house.

On the 6th of July a peasant was executed. He had pretended to be the devil and had ejected fire from his mouth, his nose, and his ears. He had appeared in this fashion to several *curés* in a wood, but from a distance, and had replied to their conjurations by threats to carry them off in the night. Some people had been frightened out of their wits, had left sums of money for him, and then fled. Nobody dared to attack him; but one day some dogs belonging to peasants hurled themselves upon him, and would have torn him to pieces if he had not been rescued. He was hanged outside the Consulat building, and immediately afterwards his head and four limbs were struck off. Doctor Honoratus Castellan, with whom I had dined, took me into a room where there were several ladies and gentlemen, and there I saw the execution from a window.

On the 14th of August the Lord of Morenholtz departed. His lackey had for a long time suffered from a persistent sore on his big toe. As it would not heal, and gangrene was attacking the bone, Maître Michel Heroard cauterized it with a hot iron. The fellow yelled in a disgraceful fashion during this operation, and tore my bonnet to pieces with his teeth; but after this treatment the bone fell off and the toe soon healed.

Not long afterwards Culmannus left. I took advantage of his going to write to my father. I told him that the summer had been so fierce that several people had died of sunstroke, and many others of the hot fever, and the plague was spread in the district of Toulouse. I also told him that Doctor Honoratus Castellan would be going to Paris in the autumn, and would stay there a whole year at court; which was a cause of grief to me, because he liked me, and I had profited greatly from his lessons. I added that I had myself begun to practise occasionally. I corrected my father's misconceptions about the religion of the Marans: Gilbert would be obliged to go to mass and to confess when he returned to Montpellier; for though the Marans had retained many of the practices of Judaism, they nevertheless considered the mass highly important, and inclined rather more to the Virgin Mary than they did to Christ. Catalan had mass said regularly for his sons, to keep them from harm. He asked me one day if the Lutherans believed in Jesus Christ, and then I told him what our religion was. 'If I were rich, I should consider my salvation,' he said, 'but as I am not, if I can but leave my children enough money to have plenty of masses said for me, I shall be happy.' He liked to repeat '*Noli venerari fratri tuo, sed alieno*', a maxim that the Marans still follow among themselves. He was an excellent man, with a great affection for me.

On the 14th Petrus Millerus arrived from Germany, and on the 23rd Sigismond Rott, from Strasbourg, later a physician in that town; with him came Johann Wachtel, also of Strasbourg. The latter was studying pharmacy, and found a place as assistant to Catalan, paying something for his keep. He told us how a gentleman called Erasmus Bucklin had been murdered some weeks before in front of the cathedral in Strasbourg, by his steward, one Onophrion Beck, who had fled to Mulhouse, where he remained unmolested until his death.

On the 26th of August Sigismond Weisel arrived in Montpellier. He was a very good shot, and his dog Faisan would search in the water for the game he had killed. He had consumed all his money, and as he no longer received anything from home, he was reduced to eating herons and other products of the chase. We Germans agreed among ourselves to contribute to his keep, even though his manners were boorish. He afterwards became a physician in Breslau, where he died quite recently.

On the 30th of August we made an excursion to the seashore with the Germans who had recently arrived, and who had not yet seen the sea. We gathered plants and shells, and bathed. Wachtel, from Strasbourg, ventured too far out, even though he could not swim, and as I was near him he seized my legs and made me swallow a lot of water. When I came to the surface, I pushed his head in turn under the water, and held it well down. When I allowed him to come up water poured from his mouth and nose, and he gasped desperately for air. He was angry with me; but that did not last.

Nicolas Cheverus, of Neuchâtel, left Montpellier on the 9th of September. He was a surgeon and had done many good offices for us Germans. He lived with another surgeon, Jean Perdris, who had relatives in Héricourt, near Montbéliard.

On the 11th of September Stephen Contzenus returned to Montpellier, bringing me a letter from Hummelius in Basel. He teased me about my projected marriage, which was already known to everyone in Basel, and praised my fiancée. He also spoke of Guillaume Hepteuring, who had been Captain Irmi's secretary and had now married his widow. Himself promoted a captain, he had left Basel with a company of *lansquenets* and had been killed in battle. My fiancée's brother Franz had been given Schoellin's daughter in marriage, together with a fine dowry. As for the physicians of Basel—Zonion had no patients, Pantaléon was in Blumers, and Hugguelin at the Margrave's court; Hubert had become a rector. Hummel added that he had great difficulty in keeping his head above water: his pharmacy was not well stocked, and few remedies were ordered. He found it difficult to believe that the practitioners were reliable: prescriptions were more often written in German than in Latin; Doctor Isaac made his own medicines for his patients, and they were diabolical preparations; all this meant that the profession of begging was worth more than that of pharmacy. The physicians knew nothing beyond how to purge with senna, liquorice root, or other drugs, and were altogether ignorant of the excellent recipes of Montpellier. So Hummel counted on my coming to change the course of medicine in Basel. This letter fired me with the notion of bringing to Basel remedies still unknown

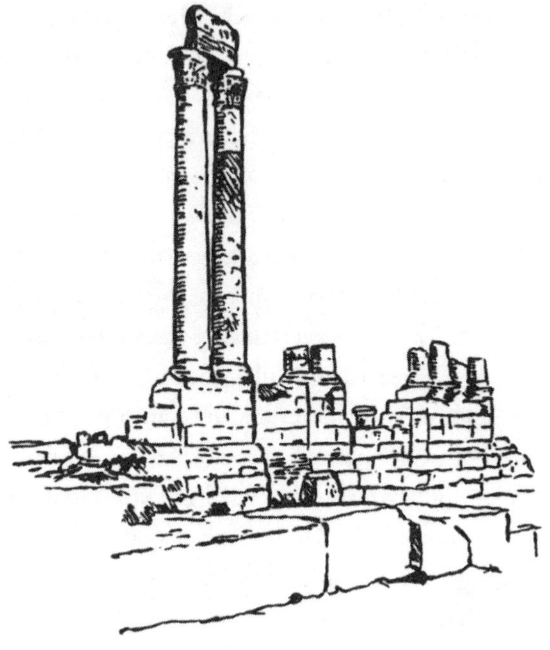

15. The two stone columns in the Roman theatre at Arles (drawing by Seán Jennett)

there, such as enemas, topiques, and other potions in daily use. With the help of God I was afterwards able to do this.

Thirteen German students formed a party to go to Marseilles. I was among them, and I hired a mule for the journey. The leader of our caravan was Contzenus, who had brought a fine horse with him from Strasbourg. The others included Wolfius, Burgauer, Rott, Chelius, Wachtel, Myconius, Lins, and the rest. Most of them were going on foot. We left Montpellier on the 15th of September, and on the first day we reached Lunel. On the following day, the 16th, we got to Saint-Gilles for dinner, and at dusk wc entered Arles, a town situated not far from the mouth of the Rhône, which must be crossed to enter the place. A village called Camargues lies on a spit of land between the two arms of the river at this point. We remained in Arles all day on the 17th and went to see Doctor François Valleriola[52] who made us welcome. He showed us his library, as well as his own writings, and some stuffed seafish, among which was an *Orbis marinus*, etc. After noting our names and recommending us to write to him often, he put himself at our service as a guide to the town. He showed us many antiquities, and among these some enormous columns,[53] made of some kind of stone aggregate, of the making of which he claimed to know the secret. There were two of them, of a very great size, at least twenty ells high, and placed one beside the other. A Roman tomb linked them at the top. He also showed us the ruins of an amphitheatre, and a building next to the church which is said to have been built with mortar mixed with goat's blood and milk. There were other ancient buildings outside the town, and in a sort of crypt a lot of white marble gravestones with Latin inscriptions.

On the 18th we dined at Saint-Martin, at a lonely inn before which there is a fountain, and afterwards went in the direction of Saint-Chamas, where we saw a gateway sixty paces thick.

On the 19th we dined at Pennes. Not long before we got there we passed through Cabanes, where we drank a wine so thick that I wrote in my notebook with it, as though with tincture of Brazil. Leaving there, we crossed a stony plain to Marseilles. As we drew near the town we heard the firing of cannon and the sound of trumpets, on account of several galleys that had just come in from

Corsica. Near the gates I saw a tree full of ripe figs—it was a good season for figs, and they were very abundant in the countryside. We lodged at the sign of the *Levrier.*

That same evening I went out to see the immense harbour, so filled with vessels that it was like a town with many towers. There was, in particular, an enormous galleon, with masts and sails of prodigious size, which had a banner with the words *Plus Ultra.*[54] It had been captured from the Spaniards, with many soldiers in it.

Next day, the 20th of September, we were joined by two Germans, Johann Mus and Philipp Kram, both belonging to Ritgrolz's company. They were superbly dressed, with Saxon breeches of a deep violet colour, from which trimmings of lace hung down nearly to the ground. After an exchange of greetings, they led us to various places, and first to the house of the Governor, the Comte de Tende, whom we saw walking in the hall with his wife by his side. She wore sleeves of linen laced with silver chains. I gave the count a letter of recommendation from Honoré Castellan. This great nobleman then made us welcome, and gave us one of his guard, an old Swiss, as a guide. This man told us that he had been for a long time in the garrison of the château Sainte-Marie, which is on a hill on the other side of the harbour, and that one night he had been attacked by the devil himself, and had put him to flight. People still called him the 'devil-chaser'. He took us to see the fortifications on the seaward side. They were well furnished with culverin and cannon, to guard the town from the direction of the sea, and their fire carries far. One of them measured forty-eight feet long. There were others built into the wall, and which could be loaded only at the breech.

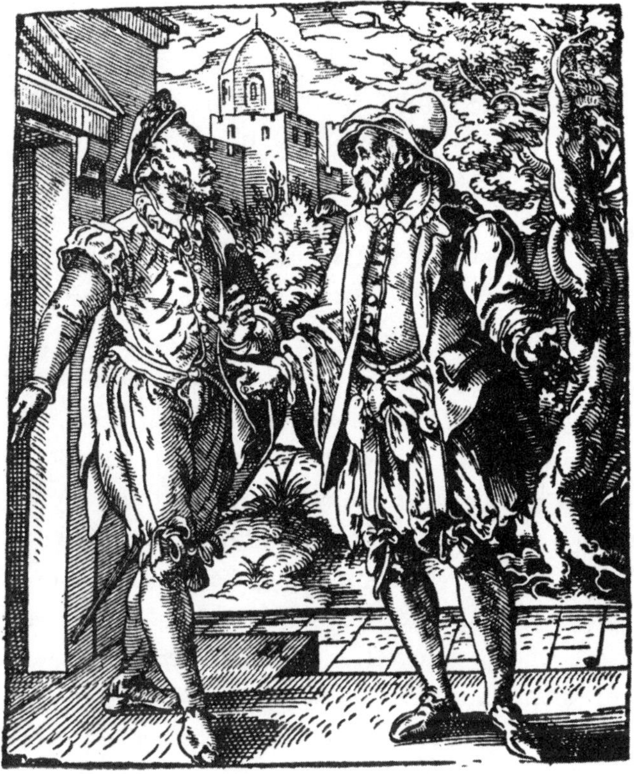

16. Two German gentlemen (woodcut from Jost Amman)

From there we went to the harbour, where there were thirty-seven galleys, as well as many other vessels. The galleys are used as prisons for the galley slaves, who are dressed in coats of red or blue wool and pointed caps. They are chained by the feet in groups of three when they are at the oars, which are many, but when the vessel is at anchor they are employed on other work in the town, principally for carrying burdens. We found some Germans among them, in particular a master armourer, who was released that day on account of the payment of a certain sum of money, and who came to dinner with us. The men carve very cleverly in wood, and especially in lentisk wood, making pretty boxes and other small objects. We bought examples of various kinds from them, and I have some of them still. However, when you go on a galley you must look to your purse. If a gift is made to them in general, they sound their trumpets, and this is taken up from galley to galley until the echoes ring.

The two German gentlemen had invited us to dine in their hotel. They were so anxious to drink with each one of us that they soon made themselves drunk. I myself was not accustomed to drinking a lot of wine, but I allowed myself to be led that day, and when I wished to go to bed I found everything spinning about me. I had to be undressed and put to bed. In the morning I felt ill until I had eaten some soup. As for our two gentlemen, they went to bed fully dressed, and in the night so watered their violet breeches that the colour was bleached out in large patches. This made me ashamed, for it was only too plain what had caused this piebald appearance.

On the following day, the 21st of September, we met in the town a physician we had known in Montpellier.

We bought some polished coral. I bought one large branch, and another unpolished, for the sum of twenty-three *batzen*. The others bought small balls, like those of a paternoster,[55] which were very cheap. The merchant also offered me, for a crown, a piece an ell long, with a crowd of branches, but unfortunately I was short of money.

Later we saw two ostriches in a yard, one white and the other black, and so tall that I could scarcely reach as high as their heads. They ate voraciously, but would not touch the key that I threw to them. We also saw rams from Barbary, with their long tails plaited—extended to their full length these tails measure at least twenty ells;[56] other rams with huge curving horns and wool reaching down to the ground; and a negro who lifted ponderous blocks of stone and let them fall on his head and his shoulders.

There are many Turks in the town, and soldiers armed with halberds and arquebuses, who accompany the Governor on his journeys.

In the afternoon we visited the galleys to see the cannon, the bridge where the troops are kept, and the galley slaves chained to their oars. During this visit I withheld my water too long, and I feared that I should die of it. I was compelled to go ashore to a pharmacy, where I got relief until the retention was finished. Afterwards we went out in a boat, and after passing through the harbour entrance, which was closed by a chain, we continued for a mile upon the open sea. We would have gone as far as a château built on a rock, but several of our band became seasick, and we had to return.

We left Marseilles on Sunday the 22nd. After we had gone some distance, Sigismond Rott, who was walking, begged me to let him ride on my mule, as he was fatigued. I agreed, but as soon as he was mounted he applied both spurs and galloped ahead, leaving me to walk a league in my high boots in exhausting heat. I was furious, for it must be admitted that this joke went too far. We went through Pennes to go and sleep in Cabanes, and next day took the road for Avignon, leaving the route that we had followed in coming from Montpellier. We dined at Salon, where Nostradamus[57] lived then, who was famous for his almanacks and horoscopes. Several of us consulted him. Continuing by way of Orgon, we reached Avignon in the evening, where I had already been twice before.

We remained there all the 24th. In our inn sweet music was played for us, and a number of Jews came, as they usually do, to offer us their wares. They had everything imaginable, especially in the way of cloth and clothing. They can renew second-hand clothing so cleverly that there is always the risk of being cheated. After dinner we walked through the town, and passed through those ill-famed streets called Pont Truncat and Peyre. Women, most of them richly dressed, sat outside the houses, and called out '*Lantz hiszer haster*'. One of them even stole a biretta from one of us, and ran into a house with it. Some of our band absented themselves here, a matter that called forth some pleasantries afterwards about *la belle Champenoise* in Avignon. We also visited the shabby streets where the Jews live. One could scarcely imagine any kind of object not to be found on sale there. Old and young, everyone chaffered.

On the 25th we left Avignon and arrived in Sernhac for a morning meal, and returned there for the night after visiting the Pont du Gard, which I had seen previously. Some of us began a game, grew weary of it, and started to quarrel. Contzenus threatened to kill everyone, and Burgauwerus tried to restrain him. It was not easy to calm the tumult, and it was a long time before complete harmony was restored. Everybody blamed Contzenus, and he left us early the following morning.

On the 26th of September we slept at Lunel, and on the 27th, in the morning, we re-entered Montpellier, after an absence of thirteen days. I had spent six crowns, at the rate of forty-six *stübers* each. My mule cost me 3 *livres* 5 *sols*, at the rate of twenty *stübers* the *livre*.

Three of my compatriots and schoolfellows arrived in Montpellier from Basel on the 6th of October. They were Theophilus Bérus, Doctor Oswald's son, and Hugwald's son Oswald. They had come to study medicine. Gilbert, my master's son, had come with them as far as Lyon, but then, not feeling well, he had stayed there in the house of Catalan's brother-in-law Jean de la Sale, a Spanish physician; he remained there fifteen days.

Our three Basel men arrived with long Swiss rapiers, and in German costume—dressed like mercenaries, in fact, and with coarse manners. They brought me several letters. My father wrote to me not to have anything to do with them, because they were unpleasant fellows. He urged me again, in view of the growing number of doctors and medical students in Basel, to work with ardour and so raise myself above the common level. I must not rely on his fortune, because he was no more than an old schoolmaster, and aged; I must realize that I should have to depend on my profession for my living. This prediction proved to be entirely true, but thanks be to God everything has turned out for the best. He said that he had had to repossess the printing house that he had sold to Louis Lucius, and that after enlarging it by another room he had leased it for a year to Michel Stella, a relative of Vesalius. He had a number of boarders, among whom was Doctor Peter Gebwiler's son, as well as Albert and Charles. He added that his son in law Doctor Michel Rappenburger, had become a citizen of Basel and had married a rich woman of the Farenbuler family, and had bought back the estate of Saint-Antoine. He added that he had sounded my fiancée, but that she had answered evasively, that what should please her father should please her as well. All the same, she had shown that she was not indifferent to me. Further, my father and mother had dined in her house, and her father had dined in ours, and this was sufficient proof of their good will. Magdalena and her sister-in-law had also promised to come for an outing to Gundeldingen, where my father had some property, and there have a meal. This letter gave me the greatest satisfaction.

A letter from my mother begged me to come home soon. Another from Hummelius told me that Gilbert Catalan had quitted Basel in dudgeon, because he had been refused a mastership. He bade me beware of him. He asked me for *trochiscos de Tyro*. Pedineaus wrote to say that he had cast my horoscope, and that I should have a brilliant future. Albert Gebwiler announced that the celebrated Hellenist and poet Charles Utenhovius had become a boarder with my father, and also that a parapet on the bridge over the Rhine had given way when a crowd of people were leaning over it to watch the disentangling of some log rafts that had got caught up below—more than fifty people were drowned. A little girl, five years old, had fallen into the water when she was going to get some mustard, with her pot in one hand and the money in the other; she had been pulled out alive with the pot and the money still clutched tight.

On the 21st of October we received a message from Gilbert Catalan that he would arrive that night at his father's property at Vendargues. Several of us rode out to meet him, and we found him on the farther side of that village. He was wearing a very high pointed hat, like a cavalier's, with a cap underneath. We stayed the night there, and in the morning we came back to Montpellier. Gilbert was not very well received by his parents, and was lodged in the same house as me. We had each a private study, but we shared the same bed.

On the 1st of November Antoine, the gardener, was sent to Strasbourg yet again, by a German. I took advantage of this to write to my father and tell him not to worry on my account, for I had learned how to conduct myself. The courses had recommenced on Saint Luke's day, but there were few professors, because most of them concerned themselves more with private teaching. I had once more begun to study the illustrated works of Galen. Nothing would please me more than to pass my doctorate in Basel, and I hoped to return home in the spring of the following year. I asked permission to return by way of Toulouse and Paris, so that I might thus visit the greater part of France. Finally I thanked him for the excellence of his arrangements concerning my fiancée, for whom I felt every day a yet more lively affection, for every one praised her to me, and Gilbert had said that he thought her a jewel among girls, and had even felt an inclination towards her himself, though he did not dare to avow it. I enclosed with my letter two beautiful silk sachets filled with *cypri*, which had an exquisite scent, and two branches of coral, one for her and one for my father.

On the 2nd of November Bocaudus presided at an anatomy session in the College; the subject was a woman. On the 10th Gallotus arranged another, in secret, especially for us Germans, at which an old woman who had died of apoplexy was dissected. When the cranium and the envelope of the brain were opened, the brains burst out and ran over the face like thick starch. On the 22nd Michel Heroard, the surgeon, operated on a young canon for a varicose vein in the thigh, to prevent the formation of an abscess below it.

On the 9th of December I received a letter from my father, sending me two *livres*, and on the 10th I received another, brought by two Prussian doctors, Valerianus Fidlerus and Bartholomeus Wagnerus, whom my father recommended to me.

On the 13th of December Antoine returned, bringing me a longer letter bound in the form of a book. My father complimented me on the journey to Marseilles, on my having the esteem and affection of my professors, and on my agreeing to pass my doctorate in Basel. I must not be afraid of failing in mathematics, Doctor Bérus having declared that more attention would be paid to medicine than to mathematics. He was glad to hear that the Germans in Montpellier did not suffer because of their religion. He added that everything was going well concerning my marriage. Magdalena had declared that she wished no other husband than me. He had given one of the branches of coral and the two sachets to her father because she was too diffident to accept them herself. He asked me to find an exchange in Montpellier for the son of Sigmund, the provost of the cathedral. Hummelius also wrote to me to say that he was sending me some elks' feet; I gave them to Doctor Gilbert Heroard.

Theophilus Bérus and Oswald Hugwaldt left on the 17th of March, after a stay of two months, during which they had led so unruly a life that the latter had taken a disease in the head, and Theophilus another elsewhere.

Gilbert Catalan had borrowed money from them in Basel, promising Theophilus that he should be lodged free in his father's house, and that furthermore he should marry his sister. Neither of these two promises was fulfilled. Gilbert had not dared to tell his father about this debt. The two men borrowed seventeen crowns from Catalan and from various Germans, and left Montpellier telling Catalan that his son owed them that amount. Catalan raged against his son. Oswald, who had otherwise a good character, left for Lyon, and after studying for some time with Monsieur de Pierrelatte, he found employment as a professor at Tournon. As for Theophilus, he settled nowhere, cheated many, and went to Spain. Long afterwards he returned from Spain to Basel with a woman whom he declared to be his wife, though he told others that she was no more than his concubine. Finally it was discovered that he had stolen a hundred francs from a Pole in Paris, and he disappeared. Nothing has been heard of him since.

On the 22nd Johannes Culmannus also left for Germany. On the same day an anatomy session was held by Doctor Guichardus, and a young girl was dissected.

On, the 27th Ludovicus Hoechstetter, of Augsburg, arrived in Montpellier; he was a former boarder of my father's. With him came Melchior Rotmundt, of Rorschach, on the lake of Constance, who had studied previously with Doctor Sultzter at Basel. I wrote to the latter, to Theobald, and to Hummelius. On the 4th of

January 1556 Doctor Saporta went to the court of the King of Navarre, to Monsieur de Vendôme,[58] where he had agreed to serve three months each year in return for a pension of eight hundred francs. He advised me to defer my baccalaureate until he returned, and gave me a letter for my father.

Fredericus Rihener arrived on the same day. He did not stay long, and on his departure I accompanied him as far as Saint-Paul.

On the 6th of January the boatmen's show was given. After performing prodigious leaps, they made a lion fight with a bull of moderate size, which they had bought. They had sawn off the points of its horns. Each animal was tied by a cord to one of two posts in the middle of the arena. The lion was made savage by the pricks of lances, and began by attacking the bull, which several times repulsed him with its horns, and would perhaps have killed him if the horns had been intact. In the end the lion exhausted his adversary, leapt on its back with the lightness of a cat, buried his teeth in its flesh, and brought it down. He then held the bull motionless beneath him, without, however, being able to dispatch it, and it had to be killed.

On the 13th of January the Germans celebrated the Feast of the Kings at supper. Louis Hoechstetter and Melchior Rotmundt stayed drinking almost all the night, and when they were drunk. Hoechstetter, who had a thick beard, treated his comrade superciliously, as a beardless youth. 'You shall be the same as I am!' cried Rotmundt, and led him to a barber, where he had his beard shaved off, and stuffed inside his shirt. In the morning, Rotmundt, seeing that no one recognized Hoechstetter, rigged him out in a cloak and hat of the German fashion, and took him among our compatriots, saying that he was a newcomer who had brought us letters. He was overwhelmed with welcomes, and invited to dance at the *Salamandre*. At last, just as we were about to sit at the table, Hoechstetter threw off his cloak, and cried, 'Fools, don't you know me?' These words aroused such a burst of laughter that I, for my part, believed that I should die of it.

I took advantage of the departure of the Lyonnais merchants on the 14th to write to my father and to give him various details concerning my studies: a fine anatomy theatre had recently been built; I should already have achieved my baccalaureate if Doctor Saporta had not had to go to the court of the King of Navarre, as the letter from the professor, which I enclosed, would confirm. I also told him of the departure and the misbehaviour of Theophilus and Oswald, and of the sorrow that Gilbert Catalan caused his father, who loved me better than his own son. Catalan often walked in front of our house before daylight, and saw that my study was already lighted—a sign that I was working—while Gilbert's room was still in darkness. Again, after supper, he saw a light in my room, and none in his son's. Gilbert began to take the precaution of leaving a lighted lamp behind his window while he went dancing in the evening or slept in the morning. I added that I regretted that I had pressed our marriage projects so hard, and feared that Meister Franz might be offended by our insistence; so I begged my father to allow matters to move quietly now, and to be content with the good regard that both father and daughter had shown for me. He must convey my excuses to Meister Franz and tell him that in a year's time I should return to Basel, or that I might spend several years abroad, in travel. He should give him the short note that I enclosed, which was open so that my father might know what was in it. Before closing the letter, I described once more how much Gilbert had been attracted by my fiancée, and indeed loved her still; but soon, forgetting her and Doctor Bérus's daughter as well, he had attached himself to a girl with little beauty or fortune, with whom he was perhaps having an affair. I knew further, from Contzenus, that Gilbert had had a ring from him during his stay in Basel, and had sent it, in a little pasty, to the girl on whom he had then set his heart, but he had been sharply refused.

On the 6th an anatomy session was held in the new *Theatrum Collegii*. Two subjects were dissected at the same time, a young girl and a woman. Rondelet presided, and I took careful note of his admirable explanations.

On the 15th of February some merchants brought me a letter from my father. It was dated the 6th of January. He had had a pain in his shoulder and in his arm for twenty-two days. My fiancée impatiently awaited my return, no less than my aged mother, who feared that she should never see me again if I delayed another year before returning. As for himself, he had no greater desire than to see me marry a person so pure and good. I also received two letters from Hugwald, one dated from Lyon, and the other from Montélimar, and two others from Italy, the first from Petrus Lotichius, and the second from a companion of Morenholtz, who was in Bologna.

On the 27th of February a German called Johann Christoph, Baron de ——rnburg,[59] came to Montpellier. He claimed to have lost his money and asked us for help, promising a horse to all those who came to see him in his own country. He was welcomed at first, but soon we suspected that he was a fraud and would have nothing more to do with him. We found later that he was a goldsmith who had coined false money, and that he was sought for this.

On the 10th of March a comet appeared and was seen at Montpellier.

On the 18th Jacobus Myconius, Benedictus Burgauwer, and Stephanus Contzenus left Montpellier to take their degrees as doctors at Avignon. Afterwards they established themselves as physicians, the first in Mulhouse, the second in Schaffhouse, and the third in Bern.

On the 24th the treaty concluded between Charles V and Henri II was announced, to the sound of trumpets.

On the 1st of April Lintz left Montpellier. I wrote to my father that a year from now I should not be far from Basel. The courses at the College were going very ill, and some were quite useless, especially that of old Schyronius, the *Cancellarius Academiae*. Gilbert persisted in his scandalous conduct, foolishly dissipating money, cheating his father, and seeking to damage me, so much that he made me want to leave. Myconius had gone to Avignon to gain his doctorate, after which he would return to Basel; he had studied well and promised to be a good physician. Hugwald was in Montélimar as a tutor to young people, and Tell, the pharmacist from Basel, was there with him, after incurring many small debts in Montpellier. Theophilus was in Paris. I said that I had been made very happy by the affection my fiancée had for me. I concluded by telling him of the *privatas disputationes* that we Germans held among ourselves. They were very useful exercises. I had been the first to speak in these, and several others had followed my example. We held such an exercise every week.

On the 9th of April five Companions of Saint James arrived from Zug in Switzerland. They were Felix Fauster, Oswald Brandenberg, Thomas Stadlin, Jacob Uliman, and Caspar Fry, who had only one arm and had already been five times to Saint James of Compostella. He made these pilgrimages as a proxy for others. We gave them a good welcome. They nearly persuaded me to accompany them in order to see something of Spain, but I was discouraged by the great heat. I have since met one of them again, in Basel, at the sign of the *Wild Man*. He had returned from France, where he had been a standard-bearer, and we recalled between us remembrance of our past travels.

On the 16th of May Doctor Saporta returned from the court of the King of Navarre, and I prepared to sit for my baccalaureate. On the 28th I was promoted bachelor of medicine at the Collège Royale, with Saporta presiding at my examination. There were only the doctors of the university to argue against me: they were doctors Schyronius, Gryphius, Fontanonus, and Heroardus, assisted by the licentiates Salomon and François Feyna. The examination lasted from six o'clock in the morning until nine o'clock. Afterwards I was arrayed in a red robe to return thanks in verse, *carmine*, in which I did not omit to mention my compatriots. I recited a long discourse from memory. Then I paid eleven francs and three *sols* and I was given my diploma duly sealed at Saint-Firmin, where the seals of the university are kept under the care of Doctor Guichardus. The diploma was in the hand of Jean Sporerus, who wrote a beautiful script.

A great noble of the Low Countries arrived from that place on the 1st of June, on his way to Spain, with his wife, a Flemish countess, and his retinue. We Germans were proud that we could show the bumpkins of Montpellier a compatriot of such great beauty, for in general they see only the frightful old devotees who go on the pilgrimage to Saint James at Compostella, singing and begging on the way in order to subsist.

On the 2nd of June a fire broke out in a merchant's house on the corner of the Place Notre-Dame. Only the four walls were left standing; all the interior was consumed. The crowd was content to watch, and scarcely any of them did anything to help to extinguish the fire. These things are very different with us, where everyone is obliged to help.

On the 17th of June the nobles held a tournament to ride[60] at the ring. The horses were richly caparisoned, covered with tapestries, and ornamented with plumes of all colours.

On the 11th of June a burning wind brought such great heat that several harvesters fell dead in the fields. It lasted until the 15th. Then a storm burst, with lightning and thunder such as I have never seen or heard in all my life. Lightning struck in several places. It overthrew part of the tower of the church of Sainte-Aularie,[61] broke the altar, destroyed several statues, and split the doors at the entrance.

On the 25th there was a great hailstorm, with hailstones as large as eggs. On the 11th of July another storm brought down a steeple. The people were in consternation, for such storms are rare in this country, where there is often no rain throughout the whole of the summer. Several herdsmen were drowned in sunken lanes at the gates of the town.

I myself, returning to my lodging one night, in a heavy rainstorm, found all the streets flooded. The water was up to my knees, and I thought I was in danger of death. A rumour was put about that the 22nd of July, which was the day of the Magdalene, would be the end of the world. This increased the terror of credulous people, who took all these storms for omens.

On the 19th of June we were visited by two Strasbourgers, Jacob Rebstock, who was later chancellor to the Bishop of Basel, and Ludwig Wolf, from Renken. They came from Marseilles and had brought me a letter from Doctor Valleriola of Arles. After three days they left for Germany. I gave them a letter to my father, to tell him of my promotion to bachelor of medicine. I had received the felicitations of the Germans in Montpellier, to whom I had offered a banquet. I had already begun to practise and I exercised myself in caring for my compatriots. I asked my father to write to Monsieur Catalan, to instruct him to give me the money owed for the board of his son Jacques, so that I might buy a horse. I also wrote to Balthazar, to Hummel, and to my cousin in Strasbourg.

It was about this rime that Saporta married Jeanne de Sos, who was a Maran, as he was. She was a girl of angelic beauty who had shown herself very kind to me at the wedding of Catalan's daughter Elizabeth.

On the 3rd of July an interdiction was promulgated against the entry into the town of people coming from Arles or Marseilles, because the plague was there. The people of Montpellier were advised not to go to either of these towns.

The two Prussian doctors Valerianus and Bartholomaeus left on the 14th of July. With Theodorus Birkmann

I accompanied them as far as Chambéry. We spent all the night copying out a little book that Rondelet had given them as a souvenir, when they said farewell to him; it was entitled *De componendis medicamentis.* We also copied out an infallible recipe for making the hair grow. The two doctors regarded it as unique and a marvellous secret. We tried it at once, to make our beards grow, for we were both beardless and impatient to achieve a more imposing appearance. Every night we rubbed our faces with the precious ointment, and by this means put our pillows in a deplorable state. We did not neglect to shave from time to time, but all these efforts were entirely in vain.

On the 1st of August we were visited by Melchior Stubenhaber, of Memmingen, a gentleman who travelled for pleasure. His wide Saxon breeches, falling as far as the ground, were admired by the French. He told us that an accident had occurred at Bourges on the preceding 1st of July. Frederic, the Count Palatine, who afterwards became the archduke, had a son Herman Louis, who was studying in that town. On that day this young man, with his servants and some other Germans, went to a meadow to amuse themselves. It was on the other side of the Avaricum, a river not very wide, but very deep and running between high banks. He was in a skiff with some of his followers, and was amusing himself by throwing a duck dog into the water. As everyone leaned over to watch the animal, the boat overturned and threw them all into the river. The young duke, fifteen years old, disappeared altogether. Nicolas Judex, his tutor, reached the bank, but, not seeing his pupil there, he flung himself into the water again, found the boy and was bringing him back, when unhappily a strap of his Saxon breeches broke, and this heavy garment fell about his limbs and quite encumbered them. Both were drowned. With them also perished Jerome Reiching, of Augsburg, who had previously boarded with my father; Jean Bellocus, a Parisian; and the boatman himself. Olevianus had also sunk to the bottom, but in the face of imminent death had vowed to leave the study of law for that of theology. He kept his word, after being saved with great difficulty, and afterwards became a preacher in the celebrated school of theology in Heidelberg. The duke and the other victims were buried in the church of the Barefooted Carmelites in Bourges, and Nicolas Gisner, who later became surgeon to the Count Palatine, pronounced the funeral oration.

On the 25th of August I received a letter from my father, five octavo leaves sewn into the form of a notebook. He said that his dearest wish was to see me return the following year to Basel. My future father-in-law was showing some impatience, for many suitors, some of good family, had asked for the hand of his daughter. She herself had made my father aware, by the intermediation of an aged aunt, that she awaited my return with no less impatience. He recommended me to pray fervently for the bestowal of God's grace on me, and complimented me on having passed the first stage of my doctorate, but at the same time warned me against the sin of pride on account of my new title. It would be the greater honour to take the doctorate itself in Basel, and that would give as much pleasure to the authorities as to everyone else. If I did take my degree in France, there would always be someone to insinuate that I did not dare to face the superior school of Basel. Everyone

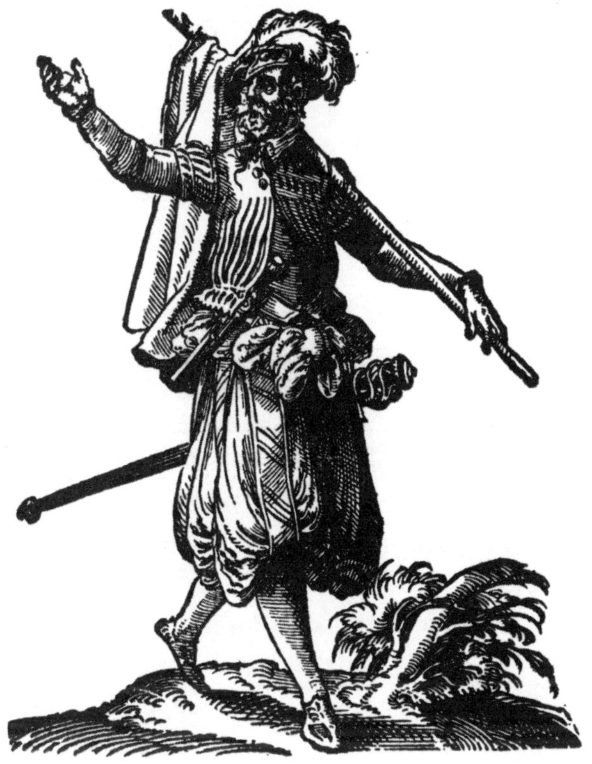

17. Wide Saxon breeches . . . (woodcut from Jost Amman)

knew the common saying about the French universities: '*Accipimus pecuniam et mittimus stultos in Germaniam*', that is to say, 'We take their money and send them back to Germany as ignorant as before'. He spoke once more of the large number of physicians in Basel, all without work, except for Doctor Huber, who spoke very well of me, and had declared at a banquet, in the presence of my future father-in-law, that I should take his place someday. The other doctors returned from Montpellier were jealous of me. He gave me the details I had asked for about the examinations and the disputations for the doctorate in Basel. No doctor from a foreign university could be allowed to practise in the town until he had sustained a debate in public, and had paid the sum of twelve florins, although the doctorate itself cost no more than twenty. My father recalled that I was a good lute player, and also that I played the spinet; music was no doubt a pleasant distraction, he said, but it must not be allowed to interfere with my studies. He added that two young doctors had committed serious blunders with purges. One had killed his patient, and the other had nearly killed himself. He advised me not to take too much risk in treating Germans, because of the penalties that were in force in Montpellier against those who practised medicine without being doctors. Such people are placed backwards on an ass, with the tail in their hands in place of a bridle, and they are led in this way through the streets, with every little ragamuffin throwing mud at them; afterwards they are expelled from the town. He told me that Count Charles of Baden had embraced the reformed religion, and had established it throughout his lands. Hilarius Cantiuncula, son of the chancellor of Ensisheim, had been drowned in the Rhine while trying to swim across it near Buken. He was a former boarder of my father's, but had left him to go to Wittenberg, to Philip Melanchthon, and afterwards to Italy, from which he had returned very learned and a good poet. My father complained of Michel Stella, a cousin of Vesalius, to whom he had let the printing house for a florin a week, and the fellow had left after thirty weeks, which meant a loss to my father of thirty florins, without counting the loss caused by Lucius, Stella's predecessor. Hummel, the pharmacist, also wrote to me that he had a son, of which I should have been godfather had I been present; in fact I became his godfather the following year. He told me that my father had bought me a beautiful lute made of cypress wood. He had thought of me on the day of the Magdalene. It was our custom on that day to eat little pasties; it was a custom that had grown up among us Germans. Each time that someone could be supposed to have intentions of marrying, we took advantage of his alleged fiancée's saint's day to make him pay for the cakes. He told me that Doctor Hugguelin had married a pretty girl named Hagenbach, with little dowry, since most of her property had already been spent to pay for his studies. He was in acute financial distress, and on top of it all, his mother-in-law, although she had sold all her property, nevertheless fell to his charge. Zonion had lost his aged cousin, and had taken the place of Doctor Michel Parisius at Mulhouse, Parisius having gone to Schlestadt. Bopp had married a Gleschter. The letter also contained some words from Doctor Sulzerus and from *dominus Castalius*.

Myconius told me of Doctor Wenticum's marriage to one of Doctor Isaac's sisters, the widow of the magistrate Israel Enhenberger, who had died of apoplexy in the council chamber. Emmanuel Bomhart, the innkeeper of the *Crown*, a former school friend, after having been refused the hand of my fiancée, had married a girl called Wachter, from Mulhouse; she was both beautiful and rich. Myconius twitted me on my having made an anagram on my fiancée, under the name of Eldam Uchmomon, which I had called my *terminus studiorum*. The syndic of the guilds, Blaise Scholly, had been made destitute on account of malversations in the *seigneurie*. He concluded with regards to Johann Vogelsang, who had lived a long time in Montpellier.

I also received a few words from Schoenauer, who sent some strings for my lute, with sly pleasantries about the beautiful Helen who awaited me in Greece. He sent me good wishes from Daniel Tossanus, then a boarder with my father, who afterwards became celebrated as a theologian.

Contzenus from Avignon, Hugwaldus, now a tutor in Montélimar, and Tellen, a pharmacist in the same town, all sent me congratulations on my baccalaureate.

On the 6th of September, a vine worker, tipping grapes into one of the great vats that they have in their *caves*, fell in himself and died asphyxiated before they could get him out.

On the 9th a man who was passing on his way to Toulouse brought me another letter from my father, dated the 20th of August. The summer had been exceptionally warm in Basel, and but for some rain that had come recently everything in the fields would have been dead. I must, my father said, be prepared to leave in the spring, because my return home was impatiently awaited. Johann Huber, who showed the greatest interest in me, never ceased to praise me. He was at the moment in Baden with his wife. My father advised me to learn to play the harp, because it was a beautiful instrument that no one knew in Basel. He had one that was very fine indeed. Daniel Tossanus wrote to me, half in Latin and half in French, to tell me how highly I was esteemed by Meister Franz, by his daughter, and by all those who knew me. He predicted that I should surpass all the other physicians, and praised

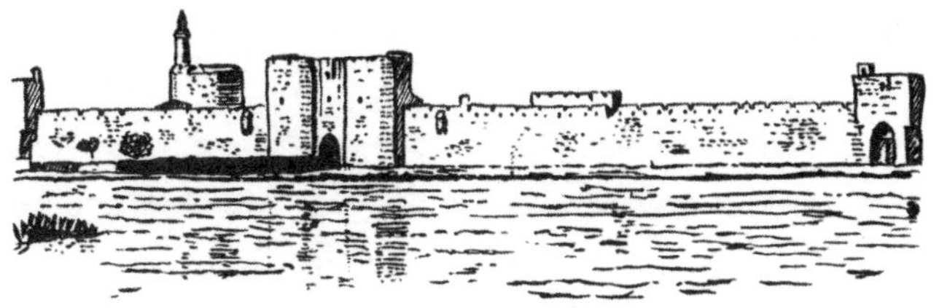

18. Aigues Mortes (drawing by Seán Jennett)

my fiancée, with whom he often talked about me, and from whom he sent me a greeting.

On the 1st of October I went on an outing to Maguelone with a number of German gentlemen—Hunno of Annenberg, Wilhelm of Stotzingen, Mathias Reiter, and Burhinus. At Villeneuve we saw grapes spread on hurdles to dry in the sun. An *étang* must be crossed to reach Maguelone itself, for it is situated on a narrow strip of land between the *étang* and the open sea. We visited the church and the bishops' tombs, and also that of the beautiful Maguelone, who is buried, so they say, in a little walled-up vault. We climbed to the platform that extends almost the whole of the length of the roof, and from which there is a view far over the sea in the direction of the coast of Africa. We were shown afterwards two neighbouring wells, one of which contained fresh water and the other salt. It was late in the evening when we returned to Montpellier.

On the 19th of October I went with some friends to Aigues Mortes. The night came upon us before we got there, and we lost ourselves, wandering about in the marshes, which were both salty and muddy. We were covered in mud, especially Melchior Rotmundt, who was wearing white breeches. It was completely dark when at last we reached the gates, only to find them closed. We were compelled to pass the night outside the walls, in a wretched inn, which nevertheless served some excellent partridges. Hoechstetter amused us constantly with his jokes, and we slept little. In the morning we explored the town and its thick encircling wall, on which we walked, the old port, and the tower on the edge of the sea, with its lantern, in which eleven persons might sit in a circle. It was used in former times as a beacon to guide vessels entering the port. We went afterwards by sea to Pérols, and returned from there on foot to Montpellier.

On the 22nd I had my first lesson on the harp. My teacher was Coiterus, a Frisian, whom I had cured of the red sickness.

On the 3rd of November I took part in the debate, in opposition, *in quodlibetariâ disputatione Salomonis, in Collegio regio*. No other German had done this since I had been in Montpellier.

On the 4th and 8th there was a masquerade, called the masquerade of the cherubim. I too put on a mask, and went to Doctor Saporta's house, where there was a ball. I took part in the dancing, and made myself known to his wife, who had asked my name; but she had recognized me some time before.

On the 18th Doctor Schyronius died at an advanced age. He had held the title of *Cancellarius universitatis*. He named his nephew Blasinus as his heir.

On the 22nd I took advantage of the departure of Catalan's father-in-law Raphael Bietz (or Biersch), who was going to Lyon, to reply to my father's long letter. I admitted that it would be no small matter to pass my doctorate at Basel, considering that I was yet scarcely twenty years old, and beardless. Nevertheless, as I had some practice in medical discussion, I might have some hope of coming through so great a test with honour when I returned in the spring. I described my method of working. I copied out good recipes that I held on behalf of Birkmann, who had got them from Doctor Georg Faber in Cologne; others came to me from Italian students—for it was our habit to exchange such things among ourselves; I wrote out *locos communes in totâ medicinâ*. I counted on returning next Easter, but it was my intention not to marry until I had become a doctor and had proved my ability as a physician. I was sure that my fiancée would share my point of view. I had made distinct progress in every department of medicine, *in praxi, chiurgiâ, theoriâ*.

In a second letter, written two days later, which this time I sent by the post as far as Lyon, I announced my resolve to return by way of Paris, in company with Theodore Birkmann, of Cologne. Monsieur Catalan had agreed to supply me with a horse and to furnish me with sufficient money for the journey to Paris; I must count upon my father to bear the charge of my return from there.

It was about this time that disturbances occurred among the students, who complained of the small number of lectures conducted by the professors. They came armed in front of the colleges, and wherever they found comrades attending lectures, they invited them to join them. Hoechstetter, who was with the Germans, came to call me while I was at a lecture of Doctor Saporta's, to whom I would not have wished to cause any distress. But Hoechstetter constantly urged me until I had to join the gathering, which was made up of students of all nations. We went to the parliament house. We elected a spokesman and he made a complaint in our name against the negligence shown by the professors, and demanded our ancient right to have two proctors authorized to withhold the salaries of professors who did not fulfil their duties as they should. The doctors too presented complaints, through a spokesmen they themselves elected. Our claims were admitted. Two proctors were named on the 25th of November, and peace returned.

Beatrice, Catalan's former servant girl, who had drawn off my boots when I had first arrived in Montpellier, was executed on the 3rd of December. She was hanged in the square, on a little gibbet that had only one arm. She had left us a year before to go into service in the house of a priest. She became pregnant, and when her child was born, she threw it into the latrine, where it was found dead. Beatrice's body was taken to the anatomy theatre, and it remained several days in the College. The womb was still swollen, for the birth of the child had occurred no more than eight days before. Afterwards the hangman came to collect the pieces, wrapped them in a sheet, and hung them on a gibbet outside the town.

On the 14th of December I received a letter from my father, dated the 15th of November. He urged me to make sure that I should not run into danger in my journey through France, and not to put him to too much expense, for he was hard pressed. He had let the printing house and two houses to Pierre Perna, an Italian, who would arrive soon from his own country. Stephen Contzenus had married a fisherman's daughter from Strasbourg, a girl called

Jung, with a good dowry. Charles, the Count of Baden, who had embraced the reform, had brought in many protestant ministers, and the Count Palatine of Heidelberg had followed his example. My father ended by recommending to me Caspar Collinus, a young man from the Vaud district, who wished to become a pharmacist. I must find a place for him with Catalan. Collinus himself wrote to me in Latin on the same matter.

About this time of the shepherds the cold was so severe that there was ice in several places outside the town. The Germans went out to skate, to the utter astonishment of the French. It was said that the Rhône was frozen near Arles.

A murderer was executed on the 14th of December. Three years earlier he had been a servant with a canon, who lived alone in his house, and carried a quantity of gold sewn into his clothes. The servant plotted with another man to kill his master. One evening, when the canon was sitting in a corner of the hearth, roasting a partridge, the servant felled him with a blow of a club on the back of the head. The villains then cut his throat and fled with the money, which came to a good sum. When the crime was discovered a sergeant was sent after them; but he allowed himself to be corrupted, and instead of arresting them he accepted a bribe and left them free to take the road to Spain. There they were too ostentatious with their wealth, and as a result they were robbed by brigands. However, the servant continued on his way, now alone. Without resources, he took employment with a Spanish shoemaker, and remained there three years. He let his beard grow, and believing that he would no longer be recognized he returned to France, and went to Lunel by way of Montpellier, but he was arrested there and brought back to Montpellier.

Although buried three years, the canon was disinterred, so that the murderer could be confronted with his victim. However, there were none of the signs they expected to see on such an occasion—as for example the opening of the wound and the gushing forth of blood; although it should be added that the corpse was very wasted. The accused man made a full confession and was condemned to the punishment they call *massarer.* He appealed to Toulouse, succeeded in escaping as he was being taken across a river, was recaptured, condemned anew to that cruel punishment, and brought back to Montpellier for the sentence to be carried out. After the judgement had been read aloud, the executioner put the man on a cart where he was laid on the lap of the executioner's wife. He then began to pinch him with red-hot tongs, and this treatment continued until they came to the canon's house. There the executioner cut off both the man's hands on a block placed on the cart for that purpose. The woman held him with his eyes blindfolded, and as each hand was cut off she pulled a pointed linen bag over the stump, from which shot a jet of blood, and tied the bag on tightly to stop the bleeding. The man was taken afterwards to the Cour du Bayle, and there he was beheaded. His body was cut in quarters, and the pieces were hung up on the olive trees outside the town.

The sergeant who had taken the bribe, and who had been betrayed by the murderer, was tied to the cart, his body bare to the waist. The executioner scourged him until the blood came, several times over. After this he was banished.

On the 11th of January 1557 there was an anatomy session in the College, at which Doctor Guichardus presided; the subject was a man.

On the 12th I put on a mask and went to dance in one of the great houses, the mistress of which possessed a doubtful reputation. We stayed there until midnight, among many other revellers. Suddenly the mistress of the house declared that she had lost a precious necklace, and caused a search to be made among the crowd. It was not found. Soon afterwards we left. My departure made me suspected of having found it, and Friar Bernhard, an Augustan monk who knew me, was commissioned to sound me discreetly on the matter. I received him in such a manner as to discourage him from coming again. I was so disgusted by this experience that I resolved not to go dancing again. The calumnies spread about me reached Catalan's ears, and he told me soon afterwards that the woman had given the necklace to a priest, and she had acted the little comedy at the ball to avoid her husband's suspicion.

On the 12th and the 14th of January I wrote to my father, sending him a box full of books, skeletons, sea fish, and all the things I had collected. I had begun my preparations for my journey home. I told him that I should be in Basel about Easter, and at the latest by the month of May. I did not delude myself about the difficulties I should meet at the beginning of my career, but I hoped, with the help of God, to surmount them all. It was my intention to introduce into Basel more effective medicines than those in use then, and to make a reputation in this way. I asked him to send money on my account to Paris. Catalan would like him to send his son Jacques back for Easter; Sigmund, the son of the cathedral provost, could accompany him, for I had found an exchange for Sigmund with a merchant, whose son would leave for Switzerland and take Sigmund's horse back with him. This was the last letter I wrote from Montpellier.

On the 18th of January a pregnant women walked on a high rope, like a tight-rope walker.

On the same day my comrades invited me to a nocturnal repast, and gave me a pasty made from a cat. I ate it, taking it for hare, but when I learned the truth, I was not too much disgusted.

On the 26th I received my last letter from my father, urging me not to delay my departure, for my prospective father-in-law was losing patience. He told me that Contzenus was established as a physician in Bern, Schoepfius in Colmar, and Myconius in Mulhouse.

I made preparations to leave with Theodore Birkmann, of Cologne, a well-educated young man whose relatives were notable printers. He played not only every stringed instrument, but also the flute, which enabled us to amuse ourselves on many occasions on the way. I bought a horse from a gentleman called Guillaume de Sandre, who was one of my neighbours; he had got it from Wachtel, who had brought it from Strasbourg; it was a strong beast, docile, and of good appearance. Birkmann also bought one. I sold my best lute, with very great regret. On the 24th of February we gave our friends a farewell dinner at the inn.[62] Afterwards I took leave of the professors, of my friends, and of some girls I knew.

Finally, on the 27th of February, I took leave of my Master Catalan. He wept freely, as did his wife Eléonore and all the people of the house. The Germans who were to accompany me part of the way arrived with Birkmann and Gilbert. I mounted my horse, in the name of God, and with a heavy heart quitted this beloved town, in which I had lived for so long. Our party formed quite a cavalcade as we passed through the gate.

We ate dinner at Fabrègues, and as night fell we reached the little village of Loupian, after a journey of four leagues.

Gilbert, Rott, and Wachtel decided to accompany us still further.

3

RETURN HOME TO BASEL

We arrived in Béziers in the afternoon of the following day, after a march of six miles, by way of Saint-Thibéry. It was Sunday before Shrove Tuesday. I announced my arrival to the young merchant who had married my master's daughter Isabelle, and then we went to a hostelry. We had not had time to be seated there before a joyous masquerade of young men and young women arrived, with music. They unmasked, and we recognized Isabelle's husband, with his sisters and other members of his family. After we had danced together they led us to their house by way of all the streets of the town, where we were shown, among other curiosities, a very ancient statue of marble. Isabelle's father-in-law gave us a superb banquet, at which a number of ladies were present.

After the meal a fire was lit in the hearth because of the cold. I found myself alone for a while with a young lady who wore pantaloons of yellow silk, and who asked me, playfully, why I must definitely return to my country and desert the maidens of France. During this, Gilbert was dancing with his cousins, and my companions from Strasbourg likewise. That evening, I remember, I broke a piece off a tooth, which alarmed me and made me fear similar accidents in the future. We spent that night in the house.

In the morning, the 1st of March, we took leave of our hosts. Gilbert remained with his relatives, while the rest of us left for Narbonne, where we arrived about midday. We had to give our names and quality before being allowed to enter. We gave ourselves for Swiss, because that nation enjoys more privileges in France than do the Germans, because of our treaties of alliance. We were led before the governor and interrogated by him, and we said that we were students who wished to see France. He did not at first believe this and sent for a man to talk to us in Latin. A letter from Basel, which by chance I had on me and which was written in that language, ended all these difficulties. My companions thus benefited by my nationality, and the governor even recommended us to an inn.[63]

While we were at table a masquerade arrived. In it was a German gentleman, who took off his mask and offered to serve as our guide. We made a tour of the ramparts and saw many antiquities built into the walls. I also remarked the height of the candles on an altar—they could be lit only from a ladder.

The 2nd of March was Shrove Tuesday, and Rott and Wachtel returned to Montpellier. Their departure filled me with sadness. In the morning, while I was still in bed, my head was filled with the thousand dangers I should undergo on so long a journey, and the thought that I should not see

Montpellier again weighed so heavily on my heart that I could not restrain the tears.

I set off once more on my journey, now alone with Birkmann. For a long time we were to find no other travelling companion. Leaving the Spanish road to Perpignan on our left, we turned right in the direction of Moux, where we had dinner. The same evening we reached Carcassonne, a town built half on a height and half on a plain, and eight leagues from Narbonne.

From the 3rd of March, Ash Wednesday, we had to renounce meat for the rest of the journey.

The roads grew worse and worse. We passed through Alzonne about midday, then Villepinte, and it had become so dark when we entered Castelnaudary that, when passing down a street to go to an inn, I hanged myself against one of the iron hooks on which butchers hang their wares. A traveller, accompanied by his servant; wished to share our supper, but then he changed his mind and did not rejoin us until afterwards. He none the less protested his desire to accompany us as far as Toulouse, and asked at what time we should leave. As this man had a suspicious manner, and the innkeeper made signs to us, we pretended that we had not yet decided. We rose in the morning before daylight, and quietly saddled our horses, so that we should be able to get well ahead, but we had scarcely left the town when the fellow caught up with us, with his servant. Both of them were well armed, though without pistols, for that weapon was then forbidden. Our situation was not reassuring. However, we resolved to leave them by taking some side road, so we pretended, as we approached a forest, that we had forgotten something at the inn, and turned back at once, promising to return soon.

As soon as we were out of sight we threw ourselves into the thickest part of the undergrowth, and trembled there lest we should be discovered. After a while we rode off, without knowing our way, and we ended by arriving at Baziėges, by way of Villefranche and Villenouvelle.

After midday we got back on to the road to Toulouse, which goes through a wood. Snow was falling lightly, a novelty for people coming from Montpellier.

As we rode along we came upon a pedestrian, ill dressed, holding a dog on a leash, and carrying a sword over his shoulder. He was singing a German song. We greeted him in the same language. As soon as he knew that I was from Basel, he asked if I knew the schoolmaster Thomas Platter. 'I am his son,' I said, 'What!' he cried. 'You are little Felix, whom I saw in his house! How you have grown!' He told us that he was Samuel Hertenstein, the son of Doctor Hertenstein of Lucerne, who later became a minister and went into the Palatinate. Samuel had studied medicine himself, but without qualifying. He had practised for a long time in Toulouse and had saved money and earned some renown there, but some months ago he had gone to Piedmont, and there he had suffered losses. Now he was on his way back to Toulouse, in the hope of earning enough in that town to allow him to return home. We continued together on the road. When we came to the hamlet of Castanet, not far from the town, and went into the inn, the host recognized him at once, and bade him welcome, calling him 'Monsieur le Docteur'. Samuel called for wine, and paid for it, notwithstanding that he had little money. When we entered Toulouse, at every step he met people he knew, and who greeted him. He even drew his sword against some, though in jest only. He was equally well known at the sign of *Saint-Pierre*, where he took us to lodge with him.

On the following day, the 5th of March, we toured the town, including the walls and the churches. In one of the churches we were shown twelve silver caskets containing relics of the Twelve Apostles. The Companions of Saint James of Compostella come to see them as they pass on their way, for here also is the body of that saint, his head alone being in Galicia. From this fact comes their song:

> They writings say, my friends,
> We must go a thousand miles
> to a city called Toulouse
> Where the Twelve Apostles rest
> and smell as sweet as roses.

Above the door into the crypt is this inscription:

> *Omnia si lustres alienae climata terrae*
> *Non est in toto sanctior orbe locus*[64]

We also saw a pagan temple, the *Tempulus Isidis*, paved with little cubic stones, no larger than dice, and as brilliant as gold. It is said that if any of these stones is covered with earth, it will rise to the surface during the night.

A curiosity well worth a visit are the great windmills of the Garonne.

In a printing house I found a former employee of my father's called Thomas.

As the plague was said to be prevalent in certain parts of the town, we settled our accounts on the morrow, the 6th of March, after dinner. Hertenstein would not allow us to settle his score for him, and accompanied us as far as Fronton, where we drank a parting cup of wine. He wept as he took his leave of us. 'You are returning to your own country, and to your families,' he said, 'while I must wander wretchedly from place to place. But I shall return. I shall not remain in Toulouse. Instead, I am going to take the road to Lyon at once.' In this way he parted from us, after writing his name in my notebook. No one has heard of him since, and I have no doubt that he is dead.

In the evening we arrived in Montauban.

On the 7th, in the morning, we went to see a beautiful monastery on the bank of the Tarn, and at the gates of the town. It had a magnificent marble portal. A monk was saying mass at the altar. I had my dog Pocles with me. I had given him this name on account of an error of Sigmond Rott's. He had imagined, before he learned French, that he had only to abbreviate Latin words to be understood among Frenchmen. One day he wanted a goblet, *poculum*. '*Apporte-moi de pocles!*' he said. This set us all laughing, and I gave the name to the dog I had then, and to every one that I have had since.

My Pocles, seeing the monk before a table covered by a cloth, and appearing to drink and eat, thought he might have a share too and went and pulled the monk by the chasuble; but a sacristan fell on him at once with a stick and sent him yelping out of the door. Pocles remembered this afterwards, and never again wanted to enter a church where there was an altar covered by a cloth. When I was staying in Paris and went to visit the church of Saint-Denis, he ran off and returned alone through the town, and I found him later at my inn. Afterwards, in Basel, he would flee every time the Eucharist was given, and he saw the cloth set on the table. But he would remain quietly in the temple during the sermon. He could not be made to enter a Catholic church, and people who did not know the reason would tease me about my dog, and say that he must be a Lutheran. Several years afterwards my father took him one day into the Vaud district. He wanted to talk to a priest, who at that moment, however, was saying Mass. As soon as Pocles saw the chasuble and the cloth, he remembered Montauban and ran off at high speed. My father ran after him, to prevent him from being lost, but the wretch only went faster, believing that he was about to be thrashed with a stick. He ran away and was lost in the town, and was never found again, which caused me much sorrow.

We left Montauban after dinner to sleep at Musa (Moisac). On the 8th of March we went three leagues farther, to the village of La Magistère. Students making the tour of France claim that Donatus lived here, but they are confounding the names of the two villages Musa and Magistère, which are neighbours. I recall that I saw cows there, the first for a very long time. In the afternoon we came to Agen, a commercial town where many Italian merchants live. As we entered a monk approached us and asked us if we had come to see the celebrated Julius Scaliger, who lived in the town. We perceived that he spoke in mockery and refrained from visiting the philosopher.

Beyond Agen the road was barred by the floodwaters of the Garonne; they formed an inlet that had to be crossed on a canoe that passed for a ferry. Birkmann went first, with his horse, and reached the other shore safely, but not without danger. I risked it after him, but the canoe began to make water, and my horse was terrified and leapt overboard before we had completed the crossing. I was lucky to get out of this accident unscathed, for I might easily have lost my horse and all my baggage.

When we came to Port Sainte-Marie and to Aiguillon we had to swear that we had not been to Toulouse, because of the plague there; we affirmed that we had passed within sight of the town, and said that we were Swiss. At the inn a parrot that belonged to our host wished us welcome so distinctly that we thought the voice was human. After dinner we left for Marmande, six leagues from Agen.

On the 10th of March, after passing through Baseille, La Réole, Saint-Macaire, and Langon, by roads that were not always safe, and going with some trepidation through a wood whose name 'Cap de l'homme' was derived from the brigands that infested it, we came at dusk to Bordeaux. The gates of the town were closed and the watchman shouted to us to go and lodge in the faubourg, which we did. That evening I ate cuttlefish and spider crabs for the first time.

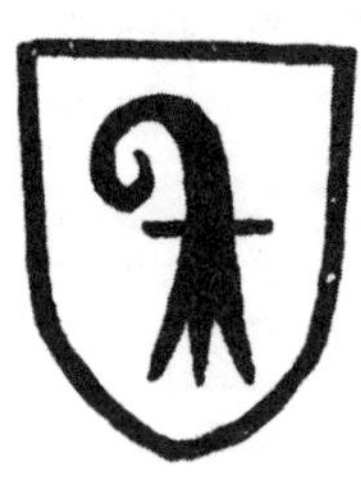

19. The crozier of Basel (drawing by Seán Jennett)

The next day we went to lodge in the town, at the *Chapeau de Cardinal.* A man from Bern, who dealt in stringed instruments, heard of our arrival and came at once to offer his services. He brought a harp and a lute to pass the time. He accompanied us during the three days we stayed in Bordeaux. We saw there how the sea withdrew, leaving all the ships high and dry, and returned in the evening. Some English ships were loading wine. We visited the parliament house, the Roman amphitheatre, and some great antique columns. We were given lampries to eat, and as we played music many people came to see us and to wish us well.

On the 14th of March we embarked our horses on board the *Aquilon* and went happily down river to Blaye. On the following day, as we left Mirambeau, we met the provost, with several horsemen, looking for some malefactors. He caught one before our eyes, tied him with a halter, and took him away with him. From Saintes the leagues became shorter. I recall that at Saint-Jean d'Angely, where we passed the night, an inhabitant of the place said to me in the street: 'You have a grand nose.' He thought that this organ was an embellishment to my face. On the 16th we slept at Thenet, and on the 17th we passed through Luzignan, where, in a beautiful park, I was shown the château in which the fairy Mélusine once lived.

We spent the 18th at Poitiers, seeing the town and the royal château. In a street I saw a bookshop with the crozier of Basel as its sign. As we left in the morning we gained a travelling companion—a piece of good fortune, for we had travelled alone since leaving Narbonne. At Montbazen on the 20th of March we were shown the château of the Marquis de Caude, and his collection of arms. Then, after a journey of eleven leagues, we entered the great city of Tours, remarkable both for its fountains and for the royal château, which we took care to visit, as well as those of Amboise and Blois. Between these two towns the road runs beside a bank of rock in which dwellings have been hollowed out. Many people live in them. When we entered Blois a woman had just thrown herself from the bridge into the Loire. She was brought out not far from us, and I jumped down to help her; but an apothecary stuffed into her mouth some tablets that she could neither swallow nor chew, and they served only to suffocate her.

On the 22nd we reached Orléans by way of Cléry, celebrated on account of the pilgrimage to Notre-Dame. We remained there from the 23rd to the 25th. There were a number of Germans in the town, of all conditions, and some of them came to keep us company at the *Lansquenet*, where we were staying. Sigismond of Andlau, an old school friend of mine from Basel, gave us a good meal, with all sorts of sweets, which gave me indigestion. I felt all the worse because the privations of Lent had weakened me.

A rumour was spread about that I was about to die, but I had recovered by dinner time, and I even went to dance in a compatriot's house, where I caused general astonishment by my skill in French dances. As we played the harp and the lute, we always had plenty of company. We were taken to see an ancient statue of the Virgin on a bridge, and to the church of Sainte-Croix, in which one may judge the exact height of Jesus Christ. There is only an ordinary ladder to climb the steeple. Some of my compatriots went up, but when I saw the streets of the town below me I was attacked by vertigo and had to descend. The Germans wrote their names in my notebook.

On the 27th, after I had renewed my saddle, we took the road for Paris in company with several Germans, going by way of Etampes, Chamarande, and Montlhéry. Before we got there we saw from afar the height of Montmartre, with the convent and the numerous windmills on it. We entered by the long Rue Saint-Jacques, and descended at the Hôtel de la Croix, opposite the *Porcelet*. There I found the Strasbourger Jocus, who afterwards became mayor of his town.

On the following day we took lodgings *en pension* at the *Sainte-Barbe*, opposite the *Mortier d'Or*, where we were given a little bedroom under the eaves. We remained here for the four and a half weeks of our stay in Paris.

In Paris I met Charles Utenhof, a young man who was very learned; and Balthasar Krugen, a kind of eccentric, who attached himself to us and would not leave us. Krugen claimed to know the whole town, had never a sou, and yet lived very well. I also met a soldier of the royal guard, at the *Mouton*, their usual rendezvous. He was the tall and imposing Joklin of Basel, who had a complaint in his thighs. With him was Fritz, from Zurich, who was married and invited us to his house for the evening.

I also went to greet Doctor Duretus and Doctor Gubillus, who were, together with Fenelius, the most celebrated physicians in the town.

King Henri II was at Villers Cotterets. We visited the Louvre, several colleges, and a number of churches, and in particular Notre-Dame, with its lead roof and its great bells. At the Pont des Orfèvres I bought a golden chain for six crowns from a compatriot; I wanted it for a present. I also bought a German testament in a bookshop; it was prettily bound and I had my fiancée's initials put on it. At the Innocents I saw a procession with so many priests and monks that it lasted nearly an hour.

One Sunday I set out to make a tour of the town, starting early in the morning, but by midday I was wearied and had to return.

I was present at the burial of a Polish noble, and also at that of a German who had died suddenly of a sore on the knee; we carried candles ornamented with a shield with his arms. I also went to the Champ Gaillard, to a street reserved for prostitutes, to see a certain Martin Bézard of Lucerne, a kind of usurer, lending money against securities, whose house was full of all sorts of objects gathered together by this means. I borrowed twelve crowns from him for my journey. He had, I remember, a habit of rubbing his nose with saliva, no doubt to get rid of a terrible scar he had there.

In April I went with several companions to Saint-Denis to see the tombs of the kings of France. On the way, there are several great statues of the saint, representing him with his severed head between his hands. We descended at the *Maure*, where we played tennis. In the morning we went to see the tombs, the most remarkable of which are those of Charles VIII and Louis XII, and that of François I, on which they were still working. The mother and the daughter of the last prince are also buried there. The tombs are numerous and very beautiful. On one there are bronze statues of a king and his queen; another is in the centre of a group of four statues, which represent women walking, as though they are about to advance towards the sarcophagus; they are very lifelike. There is also the tomb of a constable.

Among other relics we were shown a great triangular nail from Christ's cross, the head of Saint Denis encased in gold and silver, and that of Saint Benedict; a tooth from John the Baptist; the silver that Judas received for betraying his master, and the lantern that he carried at the moment of that betrayal. Among the precious objects I also saw a crucifix of solid gold, except for one arm that had been replaced with silver gilt; a cross of diamonds; a royal sceptre, on which was mounted a small unicorn's horn; another horn of the same animal, six feet long, soaking in a vessel placed behind the altar, the water being given as a drink to invalids; the gold cup of King Solomon encrusted with semi-precious stones; royal robes of every kind, and breeches and shoes. Among the antiquities were the statues of Antony and Cleopatra, another of Nero, and an elephant's tooth.

About the same time I was taken to the Tournelles, where the king's stables are. There, young pages mounted on horses and made them trot, jump, gallop, and turn in circles. The Dauphin, François, who later became king and married the Queen of Scotland, then at the French court, watched from a window. With the Dauphin was Charles, Duke of Lorraine, dressed in yellow and accompanied by all the nobles who had followed him from Paris, where he had just married King Henri's daughter. I saw the Dauphin seize a dog and throw it from a window on a page who was galloping by; the latter, even though racing at full speed, caught the beast in mid-air. Forty-five years later I recalled this incident to the Duke of Lorraine, when I was with his grace at Nancy, and he was astonished that I should still remember it.

However, I had to find a travelling companion, because Birkmann wished to stay in Paris. I found a guide who was going to Strasbourg by way of Lorraine. Our departure was fixed for the following morning, when several Basel men arrived, and among them Jacob Riedi, son of the syndic of that town, who meant to leave for Basel some days later, and entreated me to wait for him. I told my father of this delay by Bempelfort, who had been a corrector of the press in Lyon, Paris, and Basel. Unhappily Riedi put me off from one day to the next, and ended by nearly blinding himself when he had a fall during a game of tennis. He was hurt so badly that I was obliged to attend to his eye throughout the journey.

This circumstance compelled him to agree to leave on the 22nd of April. We had scarcely got outside the walls when he indicated that instead of returning directly to Basel, he wanted to visit other towns in France, and especially Orléans. I reproached him violently, and even proposed to abandon him, when the Basel guide, who was with us, made him promise that we would go no farther than that town, and would return home directly from there. So after many disputes we went once more on the paved road from Paris to Orléans, to stay again at the *Lansquenet allemand*. We left there on the 26th, and in the evening we entered the celebrated town of Bourges. There were several Germans in the hostelry, the *Bœuf couronné*, where we went to lodge. I visited the church, which is said to be the largest, and to have one of the greatest bells, in France. On one of the towers is an iron cage, in which, they say, a king was kept prisoner a long time. Behind the door there is an old and gigantic crossbow, as high as a man.

The road to Nevers not being safe, we preferred to go by Sancerre and Cosne and so towards Dijon. On the 30th we passed through Entrains, which had just been burned, to

Clamécy, on the 1st of May to Vezelay, Avallon, and Précy sur Tis; on the 2nd to Vitteau, La Chaleur, and Fleury, where I was nearly drowned while venturing along a tongue of land between two lakes; and on the 3rd we arrived early in Dijon. I hastened to see the monastery of the Carmelites, in which are the beautiful tombs of the dukes of Burgundy, and a calvary of stones with numerous statues of prostrate monks. We received a visit from young Caspar Krug, who had lived so long in this town that he had forgotten the German language. After dinner we left for Mouny; on the 4th of May we passed through Auxonne and Dôle; and on the 5th we were in Besançon, where we spent the 6th.

My companion took me to visit a family in whose house he had lived formerly, when he had come to this town to learn the French language. We talked a great deal with the daughter of the house, and we danced with her to the accompaniment of the lute. I saw her again forty-five years after, when she was decrepit and repulsive.

Several German gentlemen came to keep us company at the *Bois du Cerf*, where we lodged. They took us in the evening to some Italian merchants' shops, on the lookout for trouble, offered us a meal in their house, and then escorted us back to the inn. We continued our journey on the 7th of May, by way of Beaune and Clerval, and on the 8th we stopped at Montbeliard, at the *Tête du Maure*. There we were visited by a gentleman called Jacques Truchsès, major-domo to Count Georges, who holds court in this town. Truchsès got drunk, and persisted, despite our refusals, in accompanying us part of the way on horseback; but at the first river we came to he nearly drowned himself, and after

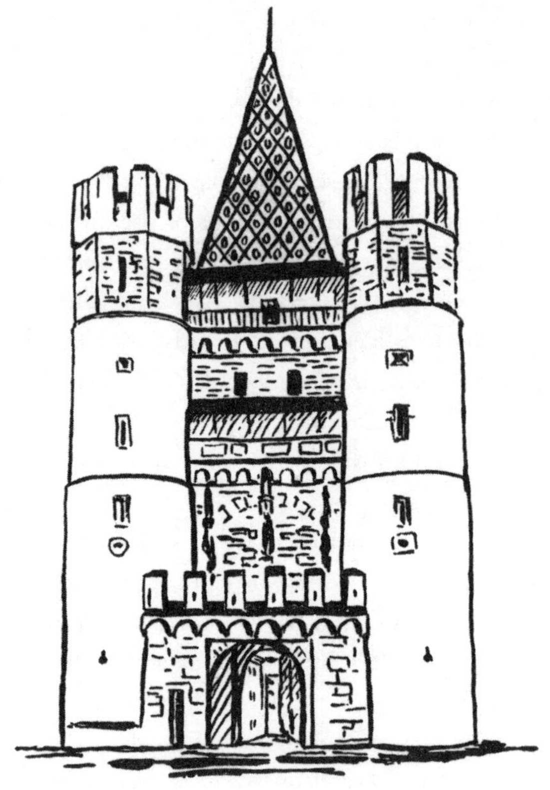

20. The Spalentor (drawing by Seán Jennett)

that he left us. We went on to Seppois, the last village in which French is spoken.

Riedi, who had annoyed me constantly throughout the journey, now picked a final quarrel with me, because I refused to lend him my cloak in place of his, which was of felt and in ribbons. I was obliged to put on a Spanish cape that I had in my bag, and which I did not want to soil. In his anger, he threatened to trail my cloak in the mud. This scene spoiled the joy of my return, and made me feel glad that I should soon be rid of this boorish companion.

But when I came in sight of Basel, and saw the two towers of the cathedral, which I had not seen for such a long time, all my troubles were forgotten. I discharged the two balls in my pistol against the door of a garden, and entered the town by the Spalen gate.[65] Riedi descended at the *Goose*, Johann, our guide, went with me as far as '*zum Gejegt*', my father's house, passing by the street of the Tanners, the square of the Carmelites, and the street of the Hospital. In front of the gate was a man going to a doctor to have his urine examined: which seemed to me a happy omen for my future as a physician. I rang the bell. The house was empty: it was Sunday afternoon. The servant was at church, my father in the country, and my mother visiting the neighbours. Soon she came running, quite breathless, and folded me in her arms, bursting into tears. I found her pale and grown older. She was wearing, as the fashion then was, a green apron with a bib above, and white shoes.

I paid my guide and gave him my cloak.

My father returned soon afterwards, with Castaleo. They both wished me welcome and found me grown much bigger. I was, in fact, a whole head taller than I had been when I left. The neighbours came in too, and the whole street celebrated my safe return.

I heard later that the servant of Dorly Becherer, the midwife, in order to be the first to tell my fiancée, had run so hard to Meister Franz's house, and had cried out so loudly, that Magdalena had been quite overcome.

My old friends, told of my arrival, hastened to come and see me. We dined together, and afterwards I went with them to the *Crown*. Magdalena saw me pass by in the street, still wearing my Spanish cape, and fled. The host, one of her rejected suitors, teased me greatly on this matter, from which I concluded that the affair was no longer a secret.

I returned afterwards to the house.

NOTES

1. The exchange system was widespread. A man from Montpellier who wished to study in Basel would seek a Bâlois who wished to study in Montpellier; each man would then live with the parents of the other without charge, so that no money was involved. This simple premise often led to considerable negotiation, as was the case with Felix Platter and Catalan.

2. Meister or Maître was used as a term of respect for qualified surgeons, as Mister still is.

3. The Emperor Charles V had to contend with numerous troubles on the borders of his heterogeneous empire. At this period Henri II of France had gained possession of Metz and Verdun, and Charles was endeavouring to recover these towns for the empire.

4. In the sixteenth century a mile was a variable quantity. Platter appears to be calculating in German miles of about 7,500 metres, equivalent to more than four English statute miles; but his ideas of distance seem to have been more often subjective than objective.

5. This refers to the remnant of the army sent to France by Edward III in 1374.

6. To be distinguished, of course, from the town of Mézieres to the north, near Charleville.

7. The River Ain then formed the boundary between Savoy and France; it was therefore at this point that Felix Platter actually entered France.

8. Rondelet was one of the most eminent professors of the School of Medicine at Montpellier.

9. Platter presumably means a protestant.

10. Henri II, whose eldest son was then eight years old.

11. An 'old wall'—the Roman theatre, which others, including a king of France, impressed by the huge façade, have referred to as a 'wall'.

12. Beside the present cemetery of Saint-Lazare, on the road to Nîmes.

13. Sugared almonds, or *dragées*, played an important part in every festival of this kind, as well as at private parties and dances. They are still a speciality of the town.

14. Catalan's pharmacy was in the Place des Cévenols, which no longer exists. It was at the point where the Rue Barralerie and the Rue Canabasserie joined, and vanished in the construction of the Rue Nationale, now the Rue Foch. It got its name from the people of the Cevennes, who gathered there on Sundays to hire themselves out for day labour. Platter witnessed such a gathering shortly after his arrival.

15. Equal to over four hundred English statute miles, or twenty-eight miles per day of actual travel.

16. 'Drap Catalan' is a term still in use to describe a material of coarse weave. A *flassada* appears to have been a woollen quilt or blanket

which could be worn as a garment in cold weather—presumably as a shawl or cloak.

17. The source of the Lez is still a tourist attraction, about fourteen kilometres from Montpellier.

18. The Fête des Rois was celebrated on Twelfth Night and is still observed in Europe, though unknown in England. A bean was hidden in a cake, which was shared among the company. The person who found the bean in his portion became king for the day and could appoint his queen. In Basel the family, or the company, must obey the king for the rest of the day; in Montpellier his privilege appears to have been to buy another cake. The bean has been replaced in Basel by a miniature image of a king; in Montpellier it may be one of various small toys or trinkets.

19. Laurent Catalan's father came from Alcolea de Cinca, in the kingdom of Aragon, and arrived in Montpellier in the early years of the sixteenth century, with his wife and son. Their true name is unknown—'Catalan' suggests the place of their origin. Laurent succeeded his father, and in 1550 sought, and was granted, letters of naturalization, so that his heirs might be assured of receiving possession of his increasing property. This Laurent was the Catalan of Felix's memoirs. His shop was then in a house owned by a bourgeois of Lyon, on the corner of the Place des Cévenols; Felix says that it was an immense house. In 1553 Catalan moved his pharmacy to his own, much smaller house on the other side of the square. The site of this was somewhere in the middle of the present Rue Foch. From this time Felix was lodged in a different house, also belonging to Catalan, which corresponded to the present façade of the Préfecture overlooking the Marché aux Fleurs, now called less picturesquely the Place Aristide Briand, and daily full of stalls selling fruit and vegetables. Laurent's son Jacques, who corresponded with Felix from Basel, succeeded his father between 1560 and 1570, and became a protestant. He achieved notability in the town, and enjoyed many honours. It was with him that Felix

Platter's brother Thomas lodged nearly forty years after Felix had left Montpellier. Jacques died about 1602 and was succeeded by his son Laurent, who became celebrated and wrote some books on pharmacy. Laurent died in 1647, leaving no sons. The fate of the pharmacy is not known.

The last Laurent had the honour of receiving in his shop the nobles who came with Louis XIII to Montpellier in 1622, when he showed them the collection of natural curiosities he had gathered during his travels. He told them that he 'would without fail have presented the collection to his majesty if the excessive quantities of powder of Cypress and of violets, angels' water, chains of musk, pomanders, censers, and such things that I prepare ordinarily, beside the medicaments of my profession, had not given some apprehension to the reverend doctors that the excess of such things would disturb his majesty's health'.

20. In the sixteenth century Montpellier had a large Jewish population. They were believed to have had their origin in north-west Africa, then called Mauretania, or the country of the Moors, and to have come by way of an inhospitable Spain to settle in the frontier towns of France-Montpellier, Béziers, Narbonne, and others. The name Maran is derived from *Maure*, or Moor, and was regarded by the Marans themselves as insulting. They had adopted the Christian religion, but retained many Jewish practices, including circumcision, which was performed in secret.

21. Like modern travellers, Platter for some time continued to think in terms of the currency of his native town. It is not possible to express the value of his coins in terms of modern currency, but it is obvious from the context whether they are of great or small worth. In general he seems to have found Languedoc inexpensive.

22. *Naveaux probably equates navettes*, or turnips. Platter does not say how he managed to eat soup with his fingers.

23. This was presumably a boat running on a line from shore to shore, as many ferries in France do. Platter's description cannot mean that some of his companions waded across, pulling the boat, for he has implied that the lagoon was too deep to be forded.

24. Four of the professors mentioned by Platter were Professors Royal, with the right to confer degrees; these were Saporta, Rondelet, Schyron, and Bocaud. Three, Guichard, Fontanon, and Griffy, were Fellows. Rondelet is the best known among them, and it was he who received Rabelais when the latter came to study medicine in Montpellier. The house in which Rondelet lived at that time still stands in the Rue de la Loge, though very much changed. Antoine Saporta is mentioned in chapter xxxiv of the third book of *Gargantua and Pantagruel* as among those who joined with Rabelais in the presentation of 'The moral comedie of him who had espoused and married a dumb wife' in Montpellier in 1531; he became an eminent physician, and was appointed Chancellor of the University in 1560. Jean Schyron, or Scurron, as Rabelais calls him (his real name was Esquiron), presided at Rabelais's baccalaureate; he was chancellor in Felix Platter's day, but by then he was an old man.

25. The College, or the Collège Royale, which was the School of Medicine, then occupied the site now occupied by the School of Pharmacy, in what was formerly the Rue de l'Université and is now the Rue de l'École de Pharmacie. The building may be the same. It was called the Collège Royale to distinguish it from the Collège de Mende and the College de Gironne close by.

26. Jacques Salomon, lord of Bonnail and Assas. He married Rondelet's eldest daughter Catherine.

27. Platter means turkeys.

28. Jean Falco, or Falcon, came from Aragon and had a house not far from Catalan's. He died in 1532.

29. Many old houses in Montpellier had terraces on the roof, or flat areas, to which people went in the evening to take the air.

30. In the deep and narrow streets of Montpellier, then and now, it would not be difficult to rig shady roofs from wall to wall to give shelter from the high sun of noon.

31. Pantaléon says: 'The German comrades make their way to the sea-shore.' Lotichius objects to the word *maris* because its first syllable is too short for the metre, and corrects to *ponti.*

32. Edward VI of England died in July 1553, still only a boy.

33. David Joris, a Dutch painter and visionary, was head of the Davidist sect. He took refuge in Basel, and lived there under the name of Johann von Binningen. His identity became known after his death and his corpse was exhumed, brought to trial, and burned in public.

34. A Dominican monastery, behind the present promenade of the Peyrou.

35. The Cour du Bayle was on the emplacement now occupied by the west wing of the Préfecture.

36. Theriaque was a medicinal treacle.

37. Zwingerus was a former boarder in the elder Platter's house, and was a professor in the University of Basel. He wrote a *Theatrum Vitae Humanae*, which was published by his son in 1642 with a biography written by Felix Platter.

38. This incident is otherwise unknown. It may concern not a sister, but a nephew of Bishop Pellicier, who was vigorously persecuted by his uncle as a Lutheran and an enemy of religion.

39. This does not imply an inn; houses in Basel were given names, which were painted over the doors, and many such names are to be seen today in Basel, especially in the old streets in the neighbourhood of the cathedral. Platter's father's house was 'zum Gejegt'—the Chase.

40. About 980 yards.

41. Peter Lotich (or Petrus Lotichius Secundus) was a Latin poet celebrated among the humanists of his day. He died at Heidelberg in 1560 at the age of thirty-two. His complete works were published in Amsterdam in 1754 and in Dresden in 1773. He fell foul of the authorities in Montpellier for having eaten meat in Lent.

42. Platter has made a mistake in the title. This book was published during Falcon's lifetime. The work concerned here was *Notabilia supra Guidonem*.

43. This monastery was on the road to Nîmes, on the left beyond the Verdanson. It was large enough, and grand enough, to lodge the king, with all his court and their followers. It was sacked by the protestants in 1562. The ruins remained until 1622, when the material was used by the protestants to build defence works.

44. Saint-Denis was a parish in the eastern part of the town called Montpellieret, on the site of one of the bastions of the present citadel. The priests of Saint-Denis lived communally, after the manner of monks. Felix Platter, a protestant, misunderstood what they were and called their presbytery a monastery.

45. Guillaume Bigot was a professor of philosophy at the University of Nîmes, and was notorious for his quarrels with the rector. The lover was a musician called Petrus Fontanus, and lodged in the same house as Bigot. The raid occurred on the 8th of June 1547. Bigot was arrested and made a poor defence against the charge of being involved in the affair. He came on several occasions perilously

near the scaffold, but was at length freed. His wife disappeared during the trial.

46. The point is obscure. Since *tunicatus* was used in classical Latin to describe the common people, who wore tunics, as distinct from the togas of their betters, perhaps the meaning here is that the girl was of common stock.

47. A quintal—about a hundred pounds in weight.

48. Felix Platter's father Thomas had been helped by the soap merchant and his wife during his youth in Munich, and in turn had given them assistance in Basel, where he found them one day in poverty.

49. The title is in Latin, *Notabilia supra Guidonem, scripta, aucta, recognita ab excell. Medicinae dilucidatore, Joan. Falcone, Montisp. Acad. decano,* etc., but the work is written in French. Falcon sent it to a friend of his in Lyon, who had promised to put it out to a competent printer—despite its university and the consequent need of printed matter, there was no printer in Montpellier before the end of the sixteenth century; but this friend was lax in his promise, and Falcon took the book back again. He next sent it to a man in Toulouse for the same purpose, but this man died soon afterwards, to be followed shortly by Falcon himself. Falcon's widow experienced some difficulty in recovering the manuscript from the man's estate, and had to go to Toulouse to get it. Returning by way of Montpellier, she was advised, according to the account, to put it into the hands of some German scholars, who would cause it to be printed in Basel; but because it was in French it was sent back to her after some months. She then negotiated with the printer Jean de Tournes, and the book was published at last in 1559—but before then the widow had died.

50. This was the name given to the pilgrims who begged their way across Europe to the shrine of Saint James of Compostella, in Galicia in northern Spain.

51. Honoré Castellan, or Du Chastel, lived in the Rue de I'Agulherie. He was one of the most brilliant professors of the school of Montpellier, and was called to Paris to become physician to Catherine de Medecis and her children. He died in 1569.

52. Valleriola was born in Montpellier in 1504 and was among the notable physicians of his day. After studying in Montpellier, he went to Valence, and lived for a long time in Arles, where he married. He was appointed to a chair in the Faculty of Turin, and died there in 1580.

53. These two columns must be the two graceful pillars that still stand on the site of the theatre in Arles, linked at the top by a fragment of entablature that might easily be mistaken for a tomb—indeed, was so mistaken, as it was also mistaken for an altar to Diana. These columns give an impression of elegance rather than of size, and Felix Platter's awe of their dimensions, like that of his brother Thomas forty years later, can only be set down to naïveté. There is also an unnecessary mystery about the stone, which appears to be nothing more recondite than variegated granite or marble. Felix was perhaps a little humourless and liable to have his leg pulled.

54. The motto of Charles V.

55. Felix probably means here a rosary made of a large kind of seed.

56. This is further evidence that Felix did not know when his leg was being pulled.

57. Michel de Nôtredame, who assumed the name of Nostradamus, had been a student in Montpellier and had gained his doctorate

there in 1529. His work during outbreaks of the plague attracted attention, and he was ultimately appointed physician to Charles IX. *Centaines*, the book of rhymed prophecies on which his reputation as an astrologer mainly rests, was not published until 1555, the year in which Felix and his friends consulted him.

58. Antoine de Bourbon, Count of Vendôme, who in 1554 had become King of Navarre. His son became King of France as Henri IV.

59. The manuscript is illegible at this point.

60. The competitors in the tournament rode at a suspended ring and sought to pierce it with a lance.

61. The church of Sainte-Aularie was in the faubourg, beside the Frères Précheurs, on the slope now occupied by the lower, southern promenade of the Peyrou. The Conseil de Ville undertook the cost of repairs, which were scarcely complete when both church and tower disappeared in the demolitions carried out by the protestants in 1561.

62. Perhaps the *Croix d'Or*, much frequented by the students. The street in which this inn stood still bears the name.

63. Lotichius and his friends had been less lucky some time before, when they had intended to go to Toulouse. They were taken for spies by the governor of Narbonne and were compelled to return to Montpellier. Narbonne was at that time on the frontier of France, Perpignan and Roussillon being part of Aragon, which was subject to Charles V.

64. 'You may travel all the countries of the world, yet nowhere stand upon such holy ground.'

65. The Spalentor still exists, substantially as Platter saw it.

BIBLIOGRAPHY

There are numerous editions of the autobiography of the elder Thomas Platter and of the journal of Felix Platter, and various selections or extracts of the journal of the younger Thomas have been published. The best of these books are given below.

THOMAS PLATTER THE ELDER

E. G. Baldinger, *Thomas Platter's Leben* (Marburg, 1793).

The Autobiography of Thomas Platter, a schoolmaster of the sixteenth century, translated from the German by the translator of Lavater's original maxims (London, 1893).

E. Fick, *La Vie de Thomas Platter, écrite par lui-meme* (Geneva, 1862).

Christian Gottlob Barth, *Thomas Platters merkwürdige Lebensgeschichte* (Stuttgart, 1886).

A. Burckhardt, *T. Platter's Briefe an seinen Sohn Felix* (Basel, 1890).

Paul Monroe, *Thomas Platter and the Educational Renaissance of the Sixteenth Century* (New York, 1904).

Horst Kohl, *Thomas Platter: Geißhirt, Seiler, Professor, Buchdrucker, Rektor* (Leipzig, 1918).

THOMAS PLATTER THE ELDER AND FELIX PLATTER

A. Fechter, *Thomas Platter und Felix Platter, zwei Autobiographien* (Basel, 1840).

H. Boos, *Thomas und Felix Platter (Thomas Platters Selbstbiographie, 1499-1552. Das Tagebuch des Felix Platters)* (Leipzig, 1879).

S. Hirzel, *Thomas und Felix Platter zur Sittengeschichte des XVI Jahrhunderts* (Leipzig, 1878).

FELIX PLATTER

Felix Platter, *De Corporis humanae structura et usa* (Basel, 1583).

Felix Platter, *Praxis Medica* (Basel, 1602).

Felix Platter, *Observationes* (Basel, 1614).

J. Fick, *Mémoires de Felix Platter, médecin Bâlois* (Geneva, 1865).

FELIX PLATTER AND THOMAS PLATTER THE YOUNGER

A. Fallot, *Le Journal des Fréres Platter, étudiants en médecine à Montpellier au XVI siècle* (Marseille, 1894).

M. Kieffer, *Félix et Thomas Platter; avec extraits relatifs à la Provence* (Marseille, 1900).

Anon., *Félix et Thomas Platter à Montpellier* (Societe des Bibliophiles, Montpellier, 1892).

THOMAS PLATTER THE YOUNGER

Description de Paris par Thomas Platter le jeune de Bâle (Mémoirs de la Societe de l'Histoire de Paris et de l'Ile de France, vol. 23; Paris, 1896).

Hans Hecht, *Thomas Platters des Jüngeren Englandfahrt im Jahre 1599* (Halle, 1929).

Clare Williams, *Thomas Platter's Travels in England* (London, 1937).

ACKNOWLEDGMENTS

I acknowledge with gratitude assistance freely given by the librarians of the University and the School of Medicine of Montpellier and the staff of the public library of Montpellier; by the Conservateur of Museums, Arles; by the librarian of the University of Basel and the staffs of the Staatsarchiv of Basel and the Kunstmuseum, Basel; and the librarian of the Wellcome Foundation, London. I also owe thanks for permission to reproduce pictures acknowledged individually in the list of illustrations.

Seán Jennett
1961

McNally Editions publishes singular, engaging works from off the beaten path. Headquartered at McNally Jackson Books in New York City, our editions are available in the US wherever fine books are sold and by subscription from mcnallyeditions.com.

1. Han Suyin, *Winter Love*
2. Penelope Mortimer, *Daddy's Gone A-Hunting*
3. David Foster Wallace, *Something to Do with Paying Attention*
4. Kay Dick, *They*
5. Margaret Kennedy, *Troy Chimneys*
6. Roy Heath, *The Murderer*
7. Manuel Puig, *Betrayed by Rita Hayworth*
8. Maxine Clair, *Rattlebone*
9. Akhil Sharma, *An Obedient Father*
10. Gavin Lambert, *The Goodby People*
11. Edmund White, *Nocturnes for the King of Naples*
12. Lion Feuchtwanger, *The Oppermanns*
13. Gary Indiana, *Rent Boy*
14. Alston Anderson, *Lover Man*
15. Michael Clune, *White Out*
16. Martha Dickinson Bianchi, *Emily Dickinson Face to Face*
17. Ursula Parrott, *Ex-Wife*
18. Margaret Kennedy, *The Feast*
19. Henry Bean, *The Nenoquich*
20. Mary Gaitskill, *The Devil's Treasure*
21. Elizabeth Mavor, *A Green Equinox*
22. Dinah Brooke, *Lord Jim at Home*
23. Phyllis Paul, *Twice Lost*
24. John Bowen, *The Girls*
25. Henry Van Dyke, *Ladies of the Rachmaninoff Eyes*
26. Duff Cooper, *Operation Heartbreak*

27. Jane Ellen Harrison, *Reminiscences of a Student's Life*
28. Robert Shaplen, *Free Love*
29. Grégoire Bouillier, *The Mystery Guest*
30. Ann Schlee, *Rhine Journey*
31. Caroline Blackwood, *The Stepdaughter*
32. Wilfrid Sheed, *Office Politics*
33. Djuna Barnes, *I Am Alien to Life*
34. Dorothy Parker, *Constant Reader*
35. E. B. White, *New York Sketches*
36. Rebecca West, *Radio Treason*
37. John Broderick, *The Pilgrimage*
38. Brigid Brophy, *The King of a Rainy Country*
39. Ariane Bankes, *The Dazzling Paget Sisters*
40. Vivek Shanbhag, *Sakina's Kiss*
41. John Gregory Dunne, *Vegas*
42. Charles Neider, *The Authentic Death of Hendry Jones*
43. Pamela Hansford Johnson, *The Unspeakable Skipton*
44. Carolivia Herron, *Thereafter Johnnie*
45. Todd Grimson, *Stainless*
46. Dinah Brooke, *Love Life of a Cheltenham Lady*
47. Kay Cicellis, *The Way to Colonos*
48. Francis King, *A Domestic Animal*
49. Felix Platter, *Beloved Son Felix*
50. Beryl Bainbridge, *An Awfully Big Adventure*
51. Philip Owens, *Picture of Nobody*
52. Philip Hensher, *Kitchen Venom*
53. Kitty Mrosovsky, *Quake*
54. Éric Rohmer, *Élisabeth*